the Hearts of a Girl

the Hearts of a Girl

of a

The Journey Through
Congenital Heart Disease & Heart Transplant

JESSICA CARMEL

New York

the Hearts of a Girl

The Journey Through Congenital Heart Disease & Heart Transplant

© 2016 JESSICA CARMEL.

Published in New York, New York, by Morgan James Publishing. Morgan James and The Entrepreneurial Publisher are trademarks of Morgan James, LLC.
www.MorganJamesPublishing.com

The Morgan James Speakers Group can bring authors to your live event. For more information or to book an event visit The Morgan James Speakers Group at
www.TheMorganJamesSpeakersGroup.com.

Shelfie

A **free** eBook edition is available
with the purchase of this print book.

CLEARLY PRINT YOUR NAME ABOVE IN UPPER CASE

Instructions to claim your free eBook edition:
1. Download the Shelfie app for Android or iOS
2. Write your name in **UPPER CASE** above
3. Use the Shelfie app to submit a photo
4. Download your eBook to any device

ISBN 978-1-63047-755-4 paperback
ISBN 978-1-63047-756-1 eBook
ISBN 978-1-63047-757-8 case laminate
Library of Congress Control Number:
2015913977

Cover Design by:
Rachel Lopez
www.r2cdesign.com

Interior Design by:
Bonnie Bushman
The Whole Caboodle Graphic Design

In an effort to support local communities and raise awareness and funds, Morgan James Publishing donates a percentage of all book sales for the life of each book to Habitat for Humanity Peninsula and Greater Williamsburg.

Get involved today, visit
www.MorganJamesBuilds.com

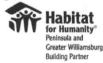

Peninsula and
Greater Williamsburg
Building Partner

Dedication

For my mom and sister, without whom I would not have survived. I love you to the ends of the Earth. To my very supportive dad, brothers and my dear friends. To Annie and Papa who, although they may not be here, I have always felt their unconditional love and guidance. Grandma Sally, a special thank you for your love, generosity and a steady supply of coffee while this book was being written...that was A LOT of coffee!

Love Always.

Contents

Prologue

"Holding to my cradle from the start,
But now my hand is open,
Now my hand is ready for my heart"
By Laura Nyro, **Timer**

I had written a prologue for this book prior to reading it. After all, I knew the story…I lived it, or had I. Helping Jessica edit this book has been both a joy and a challenge. It is amazing that my little girl, a real miracle child, is all grown up and is learning to tell her story in the hope of giving others hope. The challenge is not in the editing, but in the reliving of the often painful details of events that spanned thirty years.

Recently, I was at my gynecologist's (ob/gyne) office for a routine visit. She was late because of a baby who couldn't wait to be born! While talking, she asked me how Jessica was doing, something she always did. I told her that Jessica was well and for some odd reason I asked her if she had ever delivered a baby with hypo-plastic left heart syndrome. She looked at me rather sheepishly (I thought) and said 'no.' Then I asked her why not?

She then told me that the condition was considered 'lethal' and that the pregnancies were terminated. In that moment I knew that I was glad that I had had Jessica 30 years earlier, before the condition could be diagnosed in utero. This conversation had me thinking for weeks about how I would never have gotten to know my daughter, an amazingly strong person, a real fighter.

Jessica and Amy are the true heroes in this story. It is an honor being their mother and part of a 'team' that has been pitted against one challenge after another, with more to come. We are strong for each other and for others going through similar medical challenges.

Jessica's story is a story of amazing strength, against all odds, and I trust that it will bring hope and inspiration to anyone who reads it; the moms, dads and survivors, as well as the medical professionals who continue to find new surgeries, procedures and cures for congenital heart disease. Jessie, I love you and Amy so much and I am in complete awe that you were able to sit down and write your amazing story.

– Mom.

Foreword

We first met Jessica in February of 2009 when her younger sister Amy started a fundraiser on our nascent crowdfunding platform, GiveForward, to raise money for Jessica's kidney transplant. We had no idea in that moment that this encounter would forever change the course of our lives and the course of hundreds of thousands of American lives in the years that would follow.

At that time, we were two 27-year-old first-time entrepreneurs who knew absolutely nothing about how to run an Internet startup. We had borrowed $50,000 from friends and family and launched GiveForward seven months earlier in the summer of 2008. But by winter 2009 the business was failing and we were down to our last few hundred dollars in the bank. The day Jessica's GiveForward campaign launched is the day that saved our company.

Over the course of the next thirty days Jessica's story spread like wildfire through Facebook and Twitter, ultimately raising more than $30,000 as friends, family and strangers opened up their hearts for what would become the largest single fundraiser in GiveForward's history at that time.

It wasn't long until the media picked up on this groundswell of support. The Chicago Tribune, Chicago Sun Times, CBS Radio and eventually the USA

Today all ran pieces covering the sisters' triumphant story. This is the point when things started to take hold for GiveForward.

In the months following the news coverage, hundreds of fundraisers started popping up on GiveForward to raise money for loved ones' medical expenses. People were raising tens of thousands of dollars and sending us heartfelt emails and thank you notes that would bring our entire office to tears. At a time when we were on the verge of shutting down the company, this was the glimmer of light that inspired us to keep going. Something magical was starting to happen at GiveForward and Jessica and Amy were at the very center of it.

Since Jessica and Amy first came into our lives, GiveForward has grown into the world's largest medical fundraising platform used by hundreds of thousands of people every year to raise millions of dollars for their loved ones' medical related expenses. Jessica often says that without GiveForward, she would not be here today. But the truth is, without Jessica Cowin, GiveForward would not be here either.

Jessica's story is one of courage, relentless determination and an unyielding love between a family that refused to let the system walk all over them. Through countless surgeries, ER visits, and battles with insurance companies and hospital administrators, Jessica depicts a very sobering reality of the byzantine and at times callous healthcare system that works well for those with access but turns a cold shoulder on those without. While growing up as a cardiac kid is not always pretty, in the end, Jessica reminds us that no obstacle is too big when a family rallies together and refuses to take no for answer.

Jessica has forever changed our lives for the better by giving us a sense of purpose in our everyday work. In reading this book, we hope that Jessica's story inspires you as much as it has inspired us.

Ethan Austin
Desiree Vargas Wrigley,
Co-founders of GiveForward

CHAPTER 1

Bridge Over Troubled Water

"I'll take your part when darkness comes and pain is all around
Like a bridge over troubled water, I will lay me down."
—Simon & Garfunkel

Are you sure?" my mom asked. Her concern was all over her face as I began the walk to the operating room. It was a late, unseasonably warm September day. "Yeah," I replied, without hesitation. My nurse had given me the option to walk or be wheeled down on the gurney. Usually, the patient doesn't have that choice. You are told, "Okay, it's time to go," and your transport bed is waiting just outside your hospital room.

This day, I walked, and I went as slowly as I could to prolong the short hike up to the operating floor. Off and on, the nurse held my arm to give me stability. It was an interesting parade with her on one side and my mom, father, and sister on the other, marching into the express elevator to the operating room floor. Once the doors opened again, I paused. The nurse walked out, then my family.

Finally, me, I was the last one to get off. My steps were deliberate and unhurried as we rounded the corner and stopped at the double automatic doors. The doors to surgery are always locked. The nurse had used the wall intercom to let them know we were there. With a loud "Click!" the lock unfastened and the automatic doors swung open.

I was looking down a long hallway with a pink-and-white-checkered floor, dull white walls and shiny stainless steel doors leading to a couple of different rooms to my left. Off to my right, about halfway down the hall was a small, deserted nurse's station. Just past that, the first set of stainless steel doors read "OR 1." My nurse walked past that room and into the next operating room, OR 3, to let the doctors know I was there. Just before OR 3, she stopped us and told my family that they couldn't go any further. It was time to say, "I love you." It wasn't the place for goodbyes. I never liked the word "goodbye," anyway. It seemed so final, and I couldn't bring myself to say it. I wasn't going to start now. I could feel my eyes flooding with tears as I fought to restrain them from pouring down my cheeks.

My mom and sister were overwhelmed with tears. They did their best to remain calm and strong for me, but I knew they were going to lose it as soon as I turned my back and walked in. I hugged my mom, sister, and then my father. We said as many I-love-yous as we could before the nurse came back out of the operating room. I gave my mom one last hug and told them all I would see them later. It was not "goodbye," and it was a walk to remember. Only this time it wasn't a walk down the aisle at my wedding, like it was when Nicholas Sparks wrote about it in his book *A Walk to Remember*. Instead it was a long walk down a hallway in a hospital with the hope of having another chance at life.

I followed the nurse into the operating room. She told me, "Good luck!" and turned around to leave through the stainless steel doors. I was greeted by a couple of other nurses, the anesthesiologist, and one of the surgeons who were all going to be assisting with the surgery. The lights in the room were so bright that I had to squint to see where the nurse was pointing for me to go. After I lay down, the bright, white, surgical light was the last thing I remember as it swung around to come to rest above the cold, stainless-steel operating table. A few hours earlier, I fought back tears as the nurse worked with my veins to get an IV line started. While she palpated for a good vein, she was excited to tell me that that night she was going to watch her first heart transplant being performed. It just so happened that she was going to be watching me as I received my new heart.

Now, it's your turn to spin the wheel to see what number you land on. Spin a 10 and you are that much closer to the dreamy, fairy tale ending everyone wants. Spin a 3 and you take 5 steps back. Will you choose the path of a promising career, fame, and wealth? Or will your path lead to starting a family and the white picket fence that surrounds your perfect garden?

I am not trying to trivialize real life and make it as simple as a board game that when you are done, you can go right back to the beginning and try for a more successful round. Naturally, we all face these questions and life altering decisions. It is the normal life process we all try to figure out. Some of us do it better than others and maybe some are just luckier than others. After all, how else do you define "life"? Let's see…life…Life (according to the Encarta Dictionary) "the quality that makes living animals and plants different from dead organisms. The ability to take in food, adapt to the environment, grow and reproduce". Success! I have life and sure enough, you do, too. Your choices however, leave you at any given time, with the possibility of taking three steps forward or eight steps backward. Who is going to make it home to the big house first with the man or woman of their dreams with the 2.5 kids and who will have that successful career and all the money that one could imagine? It's a winding, colorful, path and eventually you make it to the end. You might land in second or third place and, yet, your end result is still the same as the winner's. No two paths will ever be the same, but they are, again, guaranteed to make it to the same finish line. In the end, it becomes just a game and the pieces are enthusiastically placed back at start to see where the next round takes you.

Every day we spin the wheel and take our chances, face our challenges, and undergo our changes. Everyone in real life faces them and hopes to choose the right path and move forward. At least we have the chance to make our own winding and complicated paths to hopefully a life that provides us with meaning, love, and happiness. Who wants a straight shot to the end anyway? It would be ideal to spin the wheel and land on "You're getting married!" or "You won the lottery!" If all it took to be happy was a spin of the wheel on a board game, we all would do it and, in turn, the meaning of everything would be lost under the ease of attainment, satisfaction, and greed. You lose appreciation for the small things life surprises you with. This is especially true of the things that don't come with hardship, even though they may be few and far between.

There was nothing out of the ordinary with my mom's pregnancy. It was a very exciting time for my parents and grandparents. I was going to be the first grandchild and first great-grandchild for my maternal grandparents to spoil. Everyone was excited about it. My mom had morning sickness, swollen ankles, and a fast-growing belly, all very typical pregnancy symptoms. There weren't any red flags being thrown up to indicate problems throughout the nine months. Overall, it was a relatively easy pregnancy for her, and I was ahead of schedule, two weeks early. It was a mild Tuesday afternoon, about 2:00 p.m. June 7, 1983. It's a girl! "You have a healthy baby with clear lungs and a strong heartbeat," the doctor said. Only a few hours later did the doctors take a second look at me when they noticed an abnormal heart rhythm on the fetal heart monitor. It was the "Game of Life" sending me back seven spaces when I had just barely gotten to the starting line.

Becoming a new parent is supposed to be exciting. It's a time to celebrate with baby showers, presents and cake. Anyone who is becoming a parent for the first time should be happy. However, when you are told that your child might have a serious heart condition, the happiness and joy become worry and stress. The doctors told my parents, "We are going to watch her heart on a fetal heart monitor to see if the abnormal rhythm continues." Within a few hours, they took me off the heart monitor, and I was being treated as any other normal, healthy baby. The next day I was back on "heart watch" because the abnormal rhythm had reappeared. By now, my mom was getting a whole lot of mixed messages from the doctors, and she couldn't be sure which information was correct. In a matter of three days, they went from just watching my heart rhythm and there being no problems to conducting an invasive test to see what further complications were associated with my abnormal heartbeat.

There was no way of knowing that I had a heart problem in utero and there were no tests that could have served as clues to uncover any abnormalities. My mom had sonograms as needed and went for regular check-ups during her pregnancy. Unfortunately, the sonograms done early on didn't pick up any heart condition. Jump forward to 2013, and parents are able to find out if there is an abnormality with their baby's heart at 13 to 26 weeks into their pregnancy.

An echocardiogram (ECG) is a sonogram of the heart that uses a microphone-shaped device called a transducer, some very cold gel, chest leads, and a digital doppler machine that provides a cross-section image or "slice" of the beating heart. Regrettably, not all heart defects can be seen or diagnosed using this imaging method. However, there is a better chance at early detection and immediate intervention for a newborn. Only after I was born did the doctors realize that I had a heart problem. They explained to my parents that my heart had not fully developed. The official diagnosis was hypo-plastic left heart syndrome (HLHS), double outlet right ventricle (DORV). Put simply, the entire left side of my heart never developed, leaving me with only half of a functioning heart. The left side of the heart is imperative for pumping oxygen-rich blood to the rest of your body. What saved my life was that I had a fully developed aorta and pulmonary artery, both on the right side of my heart.

Normally, the aorta is attached to the left side of the heart and the pulmonary artery is a part of the right side. A normal heart has four chambers, two atria (top chambers) and two ventricles (bottom chambers). One atria and one ventricle make up the right side of the heart, and the same are mirrored on the left side. My heart was complicated, to say the least.

I know my mom questioned herself for a long time, wondering whether or not she had done anything to cause my heart to develop the way it did. The answer to that question is: there was nothing my mom could have done differently while she was pregnant to prevent the complications of this heart defect. It was an unpredicted complication that could not have been prevented no matter what variables there might have been during the first three months. It was a random event. To date, congenital heart defects are the leading birth defect among newborns in America.

It was Friday. I was three days old, and now I was about to enter my first emergency heart surgery: closed-heart with pulmonary banding to distribute the blood to the rest of my body and to restrict some of the blood to the lungs. The ambulance was going to take me thirty miles -southeast to the pediatric hospital in Chicago while my mom stayed to recover at the hospital where she had delivered me in the western suburb of Hoffman Estates. The children's hospital immediately referred my parents to a cardiologist who would follow my case.

My parents were introduced to cardiologist, Dr. Roger Cole. He was brilliant and compassionate, especially when it came to his knowledge and treatment of his patients. In his early fifties, Dr. Cole was tall and slender with grayed hair. He walked with confidence and was a very caring, understanding, and considerate doctor. He had the most gentle touch and calming ability.

CHAPTER 2

Life is a Highway

"Roads are rough this I know
I'll be there when the light comes in.
Just tell 'em we're survivors."
—Tom Cochrane

I grew up in and out of hospitals. From my earliest memories, it was always my mom and sister right there next to me at every appointment. Occasionally, my father and grandparents accompanied us to the visits, especially when the following appointments were for upcoming procedures or surgery. The majority of the time, we waited for doctors and test results that were inconclusive and failed to provide a definitive answer to a problem I was having at that particular time.

You learn quickly that the hospitals play games of their own. It is called the "hurry up and wait" game, and that happened often. My mom always tried to leave Amy and me with a good memory after these long, physically and emotionally painful, and disappointing appointments. It was her way of trying to turn the negatives of the day into something that would leave us with memories to look back on and remember the good times, the laughs, and the talks. Going out for lunch was the thing the three of us did the most. The Lincoln Park Zoo was another frequented spot after appointments, especially when the appointments didn't keep us in the office after five o'clock in the evening. These are where the real memories remain for me. My mom somehow instinctively knew what to do. Even though she might say otherwise, she was right 99% of the time. I don't know if that was just how it was to be a mom or if she had some special powers that she used. She was the one who always took care of everything.

Considering the circumstances that we dealt with, I couldn't imagine how she did it. My father and I always had the type of relationship where we didn't see eye-to-eye. I was very strong-willed and opinionated, and he was stubborn and always wished that I was healthy and physically capable of playing sports. Many of my friends were on basketball, softball and soccer teams. I would have at least tried out for the teams if I could have. Aside from being shorter than most of my friends, my cardiologists advised against any sports, especially ones where there was a high risk of blunt injury to the chest. A ball flying directly at my chest could cause some problems upon impact. I understood his feelings. He just wanted me to be able to do all the things I wanted to do, especially when it came to participating in sports. I always picked up sports quickly, and I had pretty good coordination and skill. I came to accept my physical limitations long before anyone else.

My relationship with my mom is unique and unexplainable. We have this innate way of arguing even when we agree. We are both passionate when we talk, and that is expressed in our conversations. It never fails that while we are arguing, a.k.a. agreeing, we stop and end up laughing at each other. Everyone says that they don't want to be like their parents when they grow up. We are all more like our parents than we care to admit. I will say that if I have even a little strength and ability to fight for what I feel is right, then I can certainly thank my mom for that and I will gladly accept that I got it from her.

My sister and I share a unique and special bond like the one we both share with our mom. Ever since we were little, the bond has been unbreakable. As the older sister, I would torture her like any older sibling would do. I would scrunch down and hide in the doorway of my bedroom, and when she walked past, I would pop out at her and listen to her scream and run to find mom as I sat there laughing. I once told her that she had meat on her bones and it freaked her out. She must have been three or four years old when she ran into my mom's room, threw herself up against the wall out of breath, and said "Jessica said I had meat on my bones!"

Amy always knew I had heart problems. My mom did a good job of including her, explaining my condition, and talking to her about how they needed to take care of me and look out for me when I didn't feel good. That didn't stop Amy, however, from throwing a breath-taking punch to my chest after I had gotten home from one of my surgeries. She could not have been more than two years old when she did it. I can only imagine that her immediate reaction of "Oh shit!" must have been priceless. My sister took on a caretaker role along with mom. When I think about how much she had to give up at so young an age and for so long just taking care of me, it breaks my heart. She missed school, the socially defining years of exploring who you are, going out with friends to the mall, parties, dating, and school dances. I know neither of us would change any of it, but we often wonder what it would have been like if I hadn't been sick and could have been a normal healthy kid. She was, and will always be, the most important person in my life, along with my mom, of course.

Amy was born three years after me on May 13, 1986. During the seventh month of my mom's pregnancy, the doctors were able to determine that Amy would be a healthy baby and had no signs of heart problems. Since Amy had a fully developed and normally functioning heart, it seems like it would be hard to determine that there were actual genetic causes that could explain my condition. No one else in my family had any type of major heart problem. I just got lucky. Most babies diagnosed with HLHS are deemed to be isolated cases, and it is difficult to know the exact cause of the defect or other contributing factors in the heart's development.

The chance of having another baby born with the same condition doesn't increase with subsequent pregnancies. It was, without doubt, something my mom investigated before she decided to have another baby. She would never have put another child through the surgeries and tests I had gone through if she knew there was a risk. The doctor assured my mom that having another baby was safe and there was very little chance of major heart complications.

My sister was born at home and was a healthy, happy baby. My grandmother still reminds me that when my sister was born I kept asking her and my grandfather why my mom was crying. My grandparents answered, "She is fine. She is having your sister". Supposedly, I shrugged my shoulders, grabbed the blanket off my bed, and proceeded to the middle of the hallway and decided it was the perfect place to lay down to take a nap.

Amy and I looked nothing like one another when we were younger. We had similar features, but Amy had dark brown hair and brown eyes. I had lighter brown hair and blue eyes and, for a brief time, I was actually taller than she. We were all very lucky to have had the support system we did. We could not have asked for better grandparents. They were my mom's parents and were able to help take care of Amy and me when my parents went to work.

Family was most important, and Amy and I grew up in one that was super close. We all would have done anything for each other. We were raised with that mentality. My grandma Sally and Grandpa Louis, "papa" as Amy and I called him, were avid card players. My grandma was also a great and devoted Mahjongg player. She would have games during the day while my grandfather went to see his private physical therapy clients. They both had been retired for years at that point. My grandma, a strong and independent woman, ended her career as a school assistant principal shortly before I was born. She had three kids and went back to finish her college degree after her youngest child, my aunt, was in first grade.

My grandpa was retired from his private physical therapy practice, but he still enjoyed seeing patients who had been with him for years. When not with his patients, he would play handball at the local racquet club or join his men's social group for their monthly meetings to hear guest speakers and mingle. It was one of the social events he very much enjoyed attending. My grandpa reminded me of a football player, burly and athletic. He was sociable, outspoken and tough. But, when it came to us, his grandchildren, he was the most patient, loving softy around. One time at his monthly men's group meeting, he won a Blackhawk's hockey puck for answering a sports question correctly. I happened to be home sick from school and staying at their house that day. As soon as he walked in the door he came to find me, yelling out with excitement, "Look what I won for you!" as he proudly showed me the hockey puck with the Blackhawks logo on it. I shared the same passion for sports as he did and I was so excited to see what he had. That made my day.

My grandfather was a very smart and talented physical therapist. His other secret talent was being able to hold conversations with whoever was around while he watched a game on TV, listened to another game on the radio, and read the scores of past games in the newspaper. My grandma always said he could have been a doctor if he had wanted to. But I think he knew he was meant to be a physical therapist. My great grandma, Annie, was the person I would spend the most time with when I was over at their house. She was Grandma Sally's mother and had moved in with my grandparents some fifteen years earlier. Many times, Amy and I would stay with Annie in her room when my grandparents were out of the house.

Annie was just about five feet, three inches and would always joke that she was shrinking, just as Amy and I happened to be getting bigger and growing up. Annie's hair was a mix of silver and white. She had not changed the style since the late 1950s when perfectly rounded hair and half a can of hair spray were popular. The oldest of five, she never had the opportunity to attend college but managed to finish high school and work at Brach's Candies and the National Safety Council, in Chicago, for many years. She was quiet, yet strong and resilient. She was the sweetest, most loving woman ever. Strong women run in the family, and I can see where Amy and I get it. It is one trait we are proud to accept and openly admit. I was very close to Annie and we shared a wonderfully special relationship. I would sit in her room, sharing her smaller than average loveseat that sat against the wall just past the butterfly print partition. It separated her sleeping area from her little living room space in her bedroom. We watched the game show network, and she always told me stories about how she and her sister would go shopping together and how she had met my great grandfather Joe, the love of her life, at a dance. She loved her family first and foremost, and then came game shows and chocolate. Her favorite show was "The Price is Right." I think she just had a crush on Bob Barker, the host at the time.

She stored bars of chocolate in her drawer next to the couch and every so often would reach over, open the drawer and grab a couple of pieces. Amy and I thought her drawer was magical because there always seemed to be more chocolate candy in there each time she opened it. I loved her more than words could express. She gave me silent strength and support that was engulfing. Amy would usually sit in the den with Grandma Sally. Grandma would yell, "Ma, turn back to channel 3. You changed my channel again!" Annie would respond "What? I don't know how to work this thing," and they would yell back and forth. Annie would be in her room laughing but, neither one would emerge from their rooms to see what the other was doing or saying.

Annie's real talents were in the kitchen. Her specialty was chicken bouillon soup with white rice. Often it would be rye bread with gooey melted American cheese, yellow mustard and relish. I know it does not sound like a good combination of ingredients, especially that a six year old would want eat, or anyone would want to eat for that matter, but it was the best thing ever! Amy and I loved it. Annie never learned to drive so we could never go to the grocery store or out for lunch. We learned to gamble from Grandma Sally and during the afternoons, before mom would come pick us up, the four of us would sit at the game table and play cards or tile games. I will never forget Annie asking what color her tiles were she couldn't distinguish between the red and orange tiles that were used in the game. She would look at them, make her move in the game, and suddenly say, "I am all out of tiles!" Amy, grandma and I looked at her, sighed, and under our breath would say, "She won again?" Amy and I spent a lot of time with them and I am very grateful that we had the opportunity to learn so much from our grandparents. It is where our passion for cooking developed, in their kitchen. We learned to cook rice the old fashion stovetop way, spaghetti with meat sauce, stuffed peppers, and green bean and rice casseroles.

When I was little, I decided that I never wanted to eat hamburgers or bacon ever again. The last time I ate a greasy, fast-food hamburger, I was just about five years old. Our dog Samson had been stalking me. When the opportunity presented itself, he gently removed the burger from my hand and walked away with it, proudly. I took that as a sign. I became really good at picking the meat out of the marinara sauce when we had spaghetti dinners at my grandparent's house. I didn't care too much about the meat touching my other food. Now I won't eat anything that has touched any beef, pork, or poultry foods or products that are made with those ingredients.

I was definitely a weird kid. I can still picture the Sunday family dinners at my grandparents. The table filled with salad, meat and potatoes, rice, bread and the pitcher of water, which Amy always was in charge of filling. We all had our chosen places at the dinner table. I would always sit in between mom and Annie, and Amy would be across from me next to our father. Mom and Papa took either end of the table and grandma sat between Papa and Annie. I remember sitting there every Sunday, wishing it could be like this forever. I wanted to grow up, have a family and put on Sunday dinners just like these, when I got older. It is funny and a little sad, how so many things can change. When you are a kid, you have the feeling that nothing will ever change. Amy and I still love recreating those family dinner nights occasionally, cooking everything we can. I cherish those memories so much, they are moments frozen in time, and wish I could revisit them from time to time.

I know it was hard on my grandparents, me being born with such massive medical problems. They did their best, like my mom, to give me as normal a childhood as possible, given the circumstances. I don't know any other people who are as strong as my grandparents, except maybe for my mom. And she has passed same strength on to us.

CHAPTER 3

Living on a Prayer

"We've got to hold on to what we've got
it doesn't make a difference if we make it or not."
– Bon Jovi

Amy and I grew up with dogs. When I was born, our family dog, Samson, had just turned two years old. He had been my parent's spoiled baby up until my arrival. My mom says he was "free with a fill-up." As she tells it: my parents were on their way to a party and needed to stop to fill their car with gas. The gas attendant had a puppy that she was giving away and you couldn't just leave when there is an adorable puppy in need of a home. They ended up leaving with a tank of gas and a "free" husky and golden retriever puppy mix. Samson was a really good, protective and patient dog. He was never aggressive except when it came to squirrels and possums. I could be sitting with him on the floor as he chewed his bone, take it away from him mid-chew, hit him over the head with it, and he would

14

slowly get up and move away from me, so as not to get physically attacked with his own bone!

Squeaky toys were off limits for me, once the dog was found in my crib going after the one that he wanted. I thankfully was not in the crib at the time! After that happened, all squeaky toys were designated as dog toys.

I would start kindergarten in the fall of 1988. Before I did, I underwent two more heart surgeries. The first was when I was eighteen months old. That procedure was a Glenn Shunt and was done in order to allow better blood flow to my lungs. This was a palliative, or temporary, closed-heart surgery that would help to prepare me for the Fontan. Specifically, the surgery involved connecting the superior vena cava (a large, short vein that functions by returning un-oxygenated blood from the head and upper body to the lungs) to the right pulmonary artery, thus taking the blood straight to the lungs for oxygenation without going through the heart, hence the ability to "bypass" the heart completely.

In babies that are born with HLHS today, this surgery is still necessary to help correct inefficient blood flow. I had recovered relatively well from the Glenn surgery. Another surgery wasn't brought up for at least the next three years. Just before my fifth birthday, the doctors talked to my parents about completing the last stage in the Fontan procedure. The third surgery would be my first open-heart, and the third in the Fontan procedure series. Going into the second surgery, there were mixed messages as to what was going to be repaired in the Fontan. My mom was uneasy about the information she was receiving from the surgeons and requested we get a second opinion. Dr. Cole had agreed that it would be beneficial if it would make my parents feel better, and he arranged one for us at the Mayo Clinic in Rochester, Minnesota. When people hear "Mayo Clinic" their facial expression often becomes sad. Many responses are, "It must be dire, if you are going to Mayo." The hospital had a well-regarded reputation and was known for its state-of-the-art facilities and the care of top doctors in their professional fields.

Within a few days of seeing Dr. Cole my mom, father, grandpa, sister and I were on our way to Minnesota. Three adults listening to Raffi, a children's singer and entertainer, for six hours could not have been fun for them. Amy and I however enjoyed singing along over and over to the songs. Amy was two years old and I was about five. My mom's first impression of Mayo Clinic when we arrived was that it was "bigger than life." It was nearly twice the size of the hospital we went to back home in Chicago. The patient and family waiting areas were massive and jam-packed with people waiting to see the doctors. The staff called people in for their appointments like clockwork. I was scheduled for three or four appointments the day we arrived. Amazingly, they were all pretty much running on time. That came with one exception.

Hospitals are notorious for their long wait times, especially when you are desperate to see the doctor. Once in the room, after a two-hour wait, the doctor comes in to talk for ten minutes and then you are on your way home three hours later and with more questions. There had to be at least one appointment that the wait was an exceptionally long one. We had been waiting a while for the cardiologist to give us the results of all the testing that was done earlier in the day.

That day's conversations with the cardiologist turned out to be surprising and distressing. As he talked to my family, he boldly stated that I would not be a candidate for a heart-lung transplant because of my prior heart surgeries. I didn't realize until many years later that that was talked about that early in my care. I just thought that trip was to meet another doctor to see what they would do differently as far as the next step in the repair of my heart. Instead, this conversation was a shock to everyone. My lungs were good and strong and it made sense that I wouldn't need a double transplant like that. You can confirm the lung capacity with my mom. Apparently, I was quite a screamer, and she would compare me to the horror movies when the girls would be screaming for their lives.

During the last appointment of the day, the cardiologist came back to explain that even though I might not be a candidate for a heart-lung transplant, at some point in time I was ONLY going to need a heart transplant. Could the doctor really predict that I would need a transplant at some point in my life? Maybe he could, but a transplant wouldn't be any time soon. The doctors at Mayo Clinic came to the conclusion that the treatment plan that my doctors back in Chicago had proposed was the best for me. Since we were assured that the doctors in Chicago would do everything they needed to, we decided that it would be done in Chicago. Surgery was scheduled for some time in July1988, nearly a month before I would start kindergarten.

The Fontan procedure helps the deoxygenated blood flow back through the veins to the lungs without passing through the heart itself. The inferior vena cava is attached to a tube that bypasses the heart and then sewn onto the pulmonary artery. It allows the heart to be less stressed and worn out as it pumps the oxygenated blood to the body. This surgery would also be the first time I would be attached to the heart-lung machine. It takes over the duty of a patient's heart function when his or her heart is stopped during surgery so the necessary repairs can be made directly on the heart. The bypass machine had its own risks, but it was the only way to provide oxygen and blood flow to the body. I don't remember the recovery at all but I do remember it didn't take long for me to get back to my normal, mischievous self.

CHAPTER 4

Don't You Forget About Me

"Will you recognize me? Call my name or walk on by"
– Simple Minds

I always loved school. I never liked missing out on field trips, projects or the best time of day, lunch with my friends. At thirteen, I had a hard time accepting that I had to miss school. Somehow, the more I missed the more I was able to cope with it.

I grew up in a relatively small town in the northern suburbs of Chicago. Since many of my friends and I had known each other since kindergarten, they always knew about my heart condition. They were very understanding and supportive. My mom always informed my teachers of my medical fragility and they made every effort to look out for me. Yet, I never felt like I was singled out because of it when it came to school. It was accepted and not questioned.

My first and second grade teacher was Mrs. Pringle. I remember one morning well into the school year; both the first and second graders sat in a circle at sharing time, as we regularly did in her class. We went around the circle and shared something about who we were or what was going on in our lives. You expect first and second graders to tell you they are going ice skating, on vacation to someplace warm, or out to dinner at their favorite restaurant, something fun. There were times when I wished I was doing those things. On this particular morning, I was sitting next to Heather who is still one of my best friends to this day. I began to share with my classmates: "I am going to be going in for a heart cath. It's a test they do on my heart to check and see if it's working okay." Okay, so I wasn't the best at explaining all the medical details, but I was in first grade! I could hear some of the kids gasp as if they had never heard of that kind of thing before. Looking back, they probably hadn't. I explained the test the best I could, but the kids were still apprehensive about whether or not I would be okay. They asked me questions about the test and hugged me, not knowing what else to do. They accepted me for me and never thought twice about it. When I was slow on the playground or had to sit out due to the extreme heat, my friends were still there and did their best to include me when I was on the sidelines.

I had always had an extreme sensitivity to really hot weather. It made me weak, sick, drained my energy and made it hard to breathe. Summers in Chicago can be brutally hot and humid, warranting occasional ozone advisories and stern heat advisories. The Weather Channel warns people with heart problems and the elderly to stay in an air-conditioned building. At the time, my school did not have air conditioning.

It is hard enough for healthy kids to focus in school when it is hot. During the end of the school year, I often got sick due to the heat in the school, and my mom had to come and pick me up early. She was fed up with my not only having to sit in a sweltering classroom but with how the other kids had to, as well. She had brought the issue of the medical necessity for me to have an air-conditioned environment to the attention of the school district superintendent. I recall having to leave my classroom to go and sit in the principal's office just to be able to catch my breath and cool off a bit. My grandma even offered to pay for an air conditioner for the classroom I was in. It would have been better than getting sent home from school every day that it was too hot for me but the superintendent refused. He told my mom, "Just keep her home on hot days." I can imagine my mom's reaction, her head steaming and her face turning red, hot with rage. Pun intended!

My mom doesn't take things lightly when it comes to my condition, especially when people are unresponsive to my medical needs. I somehow managed to get through those excessively hot days at the end of each school year. Luckily school was out by the first week of June. I finished the next three years in school without having any significant medical interference that kept me out for an extended period of time.

I felt normal, like I was just like the other kids. I was an active child and always had to be doing something. I constantly pushed my physical limits, riding my bike around the block, playing basketball in my neighbor's driveway or jumping off the back of the couch screaming and pretending I could fly. I really wanted to play on sports teams, but I was never allowed to. I didn't realize it at the time, but I could run only about halfway down the basketball court before I had to stop and catch my breath. That ruled out basketball. There was no way that I could run fast enough to make it to first base on a softball team. In addition to not physically being able to play those sports, I learned from my doctors about the effect it could have on my heart. Dr. Cole and Dr. Weigel (Dr. Cole's new partner in the practice) explained that the exertion of playing sports put too much stress on my heart. Any sport that could pose a possible blow or impact to my chest was off limits, leaving me with only a view from the sidelines.

When I got out of breath, my mom said I would stop and squat to rest. It felt like there were actual weights resting on top of my chest, and the pressure hurt. My breaths were shallow and painful, and my heart felt like it was pounding out of my chest. It took me a good ten minutes to recover from moderate exertion. So you can imagine how tough it was playing sports. I was told that squatting is a typical reaction almost an automatic response that young cardiac patients do when they are tired. Once I caught my breath, I was off again. Even with my heart the way it was, I was pretty full of energy.

After my second surgery at eighteen months old, one of the doctors told my mom, "After this surgery, she will have more energy." My mom looked at the doctor incredulously and asked, "*More* energy?"

As I got older I understood how to listen to my body to know when something was wrong. Then I knew I had to stop doing certain activities.

Eventually, I got into tennis. I loved playing it! Up until seventh grade, everything was status quo. My heart was working the best it could, and I was in good shape. I was skinny. I don't remember growing very much and was still stuck at five feet tall or so. Everyone else was going through pretty healthy growth spurts.

At the beginning of seventh grade, I started taking tennis lessons with my friend and classmate, Julie. I remember begging my mom to let me take the lessons. She hesitated…for a very long time. It was hard for her to say, "Yes," because she felt that I didn't have the stamina for an activity that was that physically demanding. I, of course, thought I was fully capable of participating and finally talked her into letting me at least try some lessons to see how I did. I think my mom had a desire at this point to feel like I was a normal twelve year old. She also knew that I was capable of knowing when I pushed myself too far. Additionally, she felt a little more at ease knowing I would be playing with a friend.

Julie knew of my medical condition and could help me get assistance in case of an emergency. My second year in junior high was steadily progressing. I had started to feel something changing, but I couldn't put my finger on exactly what it was. I wasn't feeling as good as I had been at the start of seventh grade. I began to miss more and more tennis lessons with Julie. The worst part about it was Julie and I had only just begun taking our afterschool tennis lessons. It had only been a couple of weeks at the most.

The number of school days I missed increased dramatically over the next few months, and my checkups with the cardiologist had become more frequent. After missing several weeks of tennis lessons, my mom and I stopped by the racquet club to talk to the instructor and explain. We decided it was best to hold off on classes until further notice. I was not only upset at having to take a break from tennis, I also was pissed off and quite agitated from having to wear a very itchy Holter monitor that day.

I had seen my cardiologist for a checkup earlier in the day and had left the office wearing a Holter monitor. Just hearing the word, "Holter" makes me cringe. I guess it is a useful test because it's non-invasive and gives cardiologists a lot of information about the heart in a short period of time. But I always thought the Holter was a pain in the ass.

A Holter monitor is an ambulatory electrocardiography device that records the heart's electrical activity over a 24-hour time period using leads that stick on to your skin and attach to the battery operated monitor that is small enough to fit in a coat pocket. It is able to detect abnormal heart rhythms and other abnormal electrical activity the heart may be experiencing. It is also the one thing I hate more than IVs. The leads it uses are insanely itchy. My skin is very sensitive to certain adhesives, especially the kind used on the leads for this test. They drive me nuts! I was cranky, itchy, irritated and red. I don't think I stopped expressing my disdain for this test for nearly two days after the Holter was removed. It seemed like the Holter would not be a problem since it wasn't invasive, no needles and very easy. NO. Not for me, anyway. My mom always had to remind me, "Jessica, you have been through a lot worse. What's the problem?" I would just roll my eyes and walk away. This was the worst, at least at that moment.

I had been counting the minutes and watching the clock with great dedication as the second hand ticked by, bringing me closer to the removal of the Holter. I would yell to my mom, "Can I take it off yet?" "You need to wait ten more minutes," her tone intensified by the minute. I was annoyed and, in turn, I was annoying her. She, too, couldn't wait for me to take it off! When it was finally time to end the madness, I grabbed the leads two at a time until they were all finally gone. I tore those ridiculous leads off in record time. We put the monitor in the envelope that the hospital had provided and sent it back to them so the results could be interpreted.

CHAPTER 5

I Run to You

"I run my life or is it running me
Running from my past I run too fast or too slow
When lies become the truth, that's when I run to you"
—Lady Antebellum

Just a few short months later I nearly collapsed at school. The nurse had to call my mom to come pick me up. I was sitting on the bench outside the principal's office, propped up against the wall as I waited for Mom. They called her at work, and she immediately rushed to the school. The bench happened to be situated in the main hallway where students constantly passed by. A few friends stopped to see if I was all right during passing period. I can only remember that I smiled at them as if to reassure them I was fine. I didn't have the energy to really say or do much more than that. My mom flew up the steps of the school and swung the door open as if a huge gust of wind had just entered the building. She briskly walked to the bench where I was sitting.

I could barely catch my breath. I was hunched over almost to the floor, exhausted, lightheaded and with the feeling of barely being able to lift my head. By now, more of my friends were passing through the hall and noticing me on the bench. My mom and the school nurse were talking to each other. My friends offered up well wishes, words of support and "get well soon." By the next morning, I was in Dr. Weigel's office. He was one of the friendliest doctors I had ever met. He made me feel instantly comfortable and at home but was serious about my care as his patient. He was the perfect fit for the practice. My mom contacted Dr. Weigel after the incident at school to find out what the next step for my care would be. I had no idea what was going on. I had been really out of it. On the days I didn't make it to school I was sleeping nearly twenty hours out of the day, off and on.

My mom explained what happened at school. She told them that when the nurse took my pulse and blood pressure, my heart rate was over 140 beats per minute. I didn't have anything left to say about the whole thing, I just knew something was clearly wrong, and I just wanted to feel better.

A normal heart rate, especially for a twelve-year-old kid, should be only 95 beats per minute. That is the highest it should be at rest without exertion. Dr. Weigel ordered an x-ray, among other tests, so he could determine why it had increased so much.

After many tests and doctor's visits, Dr. Cole and Dr. Weigel came to the conclusion that the only thing that could be done was another surgery to repair elements from the previous surgery (the Fontan surgery at five years old). Now, I was beginning the work-up for my fourth surgery, a revised Fontan. The doctors found that I was having episodes of tachycardia, a heart rhythm problem where the heart beats at an irregular rate and very rapid speed.

It wasn't enough that I was having medical problems, but now we were about to deal with insurance problems. At the time I was insured by an HMO. When you are desperate to see a doctor as soon as possible, HMO plans really aren't accommodating. You can't just make an appointment and go in anytime. Whenever I needed to see a doctor, get a blood test or an x-ray, I needed a referral first. Some referrals took three days to a week to process and approve.

Everything was taking so much longer to set up than it should have. In a case that was time sensitive, the HMO seemed to be taking its time processing the papers to approve the surgery. Mom was on the phone fighting back and forth with the hospital and insurance representatives just to get the referrals approved.

If you can avoid having an HMO, do it. Unless you are an exceptionally healthy person who never goes to the doctor or gets sick, it is not a great idea. It is particularly inconvenient when you are severely ill. I get that this type of insurance works for a lot of "healthy" people. For them it is far less expensive. You also get what you pay for which seems to me to be very little choice in your healthcare. After the near fainting episode at school, Dr. Weigel was looking at the x-ray he had sent me in for earlier that day. I stood right next to him and pretended to study the x-ray as if I knew what I was looking at as he proceeded to explain what he saw.

"This is your heart. A normal heart is about the size of your fist." When you are an adolescent, the size of your fist is what the size of your heart should be. The same is true for when you are an adult. He asked me to make a fist for him so I could see the approximate size my heart should be for my age. "That is pretty small, huh? Your heart is three times the size it should be," he explained. It was as clear as the x-ray, when lit by the florescent light. My heart had very little room left to be able to beat normally inside my chest; The Mediastinum is the central part of the thoracic cavity where the heart is contained. It was so enlarged that it couldn't keep up the rate at which it was pumping, and that was the reason the tachycardia episodes were growing progressively worse. The only immediate thing that could be done at this point was to monitor my heart with frequent electrocardiograms (EKGs) that check for problems with the electrical activity of the heart and echocardiograms, echoes of sound waves that create an image of the heart. Dr. Weigel always performed my echo. I would lie on my right side at the start of the test as Dr. Weigel moved the transducer around to get a better view of my poorly functioning heart. I stared at the shelves of neatly stacked VHS tapes. There was a whole wall of patient's echoes, recorded and stored for future comparisons. I asked Dr. Weigel a variety of questions during these nearly hour-long echoes. I told him about school and what fun things Mom had planned for us during the week. Often, I would talk with him during the whole test, with a few exceptions, like when he told me to, "Take a deep breath and hold it. Ok, you can breathe now."

In the midst of all these cardiac events, my parents were in the process of finalizing their divorce. They had been married for nearly sixteen years, and it wasn't working anymore. In June 1995 my father moved to an apartment just a few blocks away so it would be easy for us to see him. However, his apartment building had three flights of stairs and, at that point I wasn't able to make it up two steps before needing to be carried up the rest of the way. I was instantly out of breath and had pain in my chest. Now six months later in December 1996, I was heading in for my fourth heart surgery. I had a revised Fontan with cryoablation, which essentially translates into freezing the heart cells that were associated with the tachycardia episodes I was experiencing. A fantastic piece of equipment, a pacemaker, was also a fun addition to this surgery. Yes, I have a wicked sarcastic side and this won't be the last time I express it.

CHAPTER 6

Breath of Life

"And my heart is a hollow plain for the devil
to dance again and the room is quiet, oh."
—Florence and the Machine

This surgery was rough for everyone. In particular, Amy was having a hard time transitioning in school. She was finishing fifth grade and preparing to leave elementary to go to sixth grade at the Junior High. I was at the beginning of eighth grade, and I wasn't off to a great start.

It is important to understand that the Fontan procedure is not a cure for hypoplastic left heart syndrome (HLHS). It is merely a way to reduce the symptoms and severity of patients born with this condition. This surgical revision was going to help redirect blood flow from the inferior vena cava, the large vein that carries de-oxygenated blood from the lower half of the body back to the right side of the heart.

The episodes of tachycardia were a further sign that the heart I was born with was weakening. My doctors made the decision to put in a pacemaker in the hope it would help regulate my heart rate, which was a reflection of how hard my heart was working and how stress was affecting my heart. I was by no means thrilled with the idea of having a foreign object in my body to deal with much less dealing with the unknown of what life with a pacemaker would be like.

There are two places that the doctors can place a pacemaker. One is in the lower abdomen and the second is in the upper chest region. I didn't get to choose where I wanted the pacemaker to be placed. Had I had that choice, it would have been placed back in the sterilized surgical bag it came in. I made it through the surgery without complications and with the pacemaker located in my lower abdomen.

Depending on the way I sat, it would dig into my side and I would have to shift to a different position so it wouldn't bother me as much. I was told that I needed to be careful with cell phones because there was a chance they could deactivate the pacemaker. I couldn't have any electronic device in the vicinity. Anytime I went to the airport, the metal detectors could stop the pacemaker from working, so I needed to avoid those. There was a whole list of do's and don'ts that the nurses and doctors explained to me before I was discharged from the hospital. It was about a week or so later when I finally went home. I didn't want to be alone in my room, so I ended up staying with Amy in hers. She had separated her two bunk beds and she was nice enough to let me recover there.

I couldn't bring myself to take the bandages off my chest to let my scar "breathe." I had a bad feeling that I wasn't going to like the way it looked. It wasn't going to be good. My mom insisted that it couldn't be that bad even though she knew that the doctors had left my scar less than esthetically pleasing. It took me a couple days before I could even bring myself to look under the bandages. It looked horrible to me. I don't think I stopped crying for the rest of the week. If I looked down at it, I started crying again. It was messy and uneven. It looked like a huge worm was sewn down my chest. It was not the neat, flat and symmetrical scar I expected. It made me sick and I was more self-conscious about it than I had ever been about the scars from previous surgeries.

I found out later that Dr. Mavroudis, the surgeon who had performed my operation, talked to my mother and implied that this was only a temporary fix. He said that he had done everything he could for me, but he didn't think it was going to be enough.

My mom believed that the reason that Dr. Mavroudis left the scar so undesirable was because my chest was just going to be opened again and probably soon. He knew that this wasn't going to be my last surgery.

The next three years with the pacemaker weren't terrible, and I grew adjusted to it in about six months. I had checkups every three to six months, and they were long and tiring. The doctors also had to adjust the sensitivity level on the pacemaker from time to time. Nearly every appointment required they put in an IV to administer the medication needed to test my pacemaker's reaction to the changes in my heart rhythm. When I get IVs, I am anxious, and there is pain. I have always had problems with IVs. My veins are sizeable but they aren't easily punctured. Thus, the nurses never could get the IV started.

I remember one particular visit vividly. What happened that day, all the blood, ruined my favorite pair of jeans. The nurse was making her second attempt at putting in an IV so she could start the medicine that was used to track the pacemaker. I nearly threw up over the side of the bed because I saw blood spewing from the IV site. Blood was flowing down my arm and soaking my jeans. I couldn't reach the towels, which were sitting on the windowsill, to soak up the blood on my lap. My reaction time wasn't fast enough and my hands were full. One hand held pressure on the spot where I was bleeding while I held the bleeding arm in the air, hoping gravity would slow the surge.

Finally, I was lying down and the test was beginning. It took about a half hour to check the pacemaker, a hell of a lot less time than it took to get the IV started. The nurse held a special magnetic wand over my stomach until she heard a static sound. This let her know that she had found where the pacemaker was. Then she got a baseline read of my heart rhythm, and then determined my heart rate, and the battery life left on the pacemaker. If at any time the battery needed to be replaced, there would be a small outpatient procedure to change it.

My doctor was the head of pediatric cardiology, specializing in working with children who had pacemakers. He came in and made sure everything looked good, making adjustments if necessary. He was a really wonderful guy. He would make me laugh every time I had an appointment. He had heard about my favorite pair of jeans and that was his joke every time he came in to the room: "Did the nurse get any blood on your jeans today?" News always traveled fast when I was the patient.

On every other visit, I would go home with a Holter monitor to make sure I wasn't having any more tachycardia episodes. If I did, it monitored when the pacemaker was shocking my heart back to its normal pace. I wouldn't leave very happy with the Holter, and my doctor knew it. He always told me, "I know you are not happy with me right now, but you have to do this so we can make sure everything with your heart is stable." I tried to smile as if I accepted this, but the second I walked out of the room towards the elevator I was already in a bad mood, complaining about being itchy and about to cry again.

I didn't find the following story all that funny when it happened. I was still adjusting to living with the pacemaker, but my mom and Amy won't soon let me forget it. One of the rules my doctors gave me upon leaving the hospital was to be careful around electronic devices and strong magnetic fields. The lithium iodine battery that keeps the pacemaker working is highly sensitive. If it happened to come into contact with a cell phone or a metal detector the pacemaker could shut off. I was running up the stairs at home as I was beginning to regain some of my energy when the smoke alarm went off. I stopped dead in my tracks for a split second before running into Mom's room, completely out of breath, looking panicked, and saying, "I think my pacemaker just set off the smoke detector!" My mom didn't seem at all worried and tried to convince me otherwise. "I doubt it. I don't think your pacemaker can do that," she consoled. I was sure that it was not a coincidence, because the alarm suddenly sounded just as I passed by.

Amy heard the commotion and poked her head out of her room to see what was going on. My mom told her, "Everything is fine. Jessica just thought she set off the smoke detector." Amy smirked, and then started to really laugh at the idea. I was totally serious, but now both Amy and mom were laughing. All I could hear in my head were the doctors telling me to stay away from electronic devices, and I had instantly associated the smoke detector with one of those electronic devices! I was at least an attentive patient and this was another learning experience, a laughable one, but nonetheless informative. As far as the smoke detector goes, its batteries were dead, ironically, and needed to be changed. For the next three years, they often asked if I had set off the smoke detector lately. I was even asked by the doctor who was in charge of following my pacemaker care. Everyone eventually knew all my idiotic mishaps. Suffice it to say we all got a good laugh out of it. I still get reminded of that incident every so often, especially when the alarm goes off.

There was a lot to keep up with having the pacemaker. When I didn't go into the hospital for the pacemaker checks, I was to perform home checks. Early on I was given a small transmitter box that I could use to send the reading to the nurse. These were weekly scheduled appointments that only required a landline phone, a glass of water, and a clock with a second hand. The nurse would call from the "pacemaker hotline" and I would be ready to put the phone in position. The glass of water was for wetting my index fingers before placing the small monitors on my fingers to send the reading to the nurse. There were two sessions, each forty seconds long. The first was a baseline reading and heart rate and the second was with a magnet placed over the pacemaker to see if there were any adjustments that needed to be made to it directly. When I was finished, I picked up the phone to talk to the nurse, made sure the transmission went through and the test was complete. This simple procedure was one of the very few tests that I didn't have a problem with or attitude about doing.

CHAPTER 7

This is Love

"This is why we do it, this is worth the pain
This is where we fall down and get back up again
This is where the heart lies
This is from above
Love is this, this is love"
– The Script

The scar was still horrible, and I had no choice but to suck it up and try not to pay too much attention to it. I couldn't stand to look at the red, lumpy thing down my chest. My clothes covered as much of it as possible, but it came to rest just at the base of my neck. It was hard to cover up that much of it in warm weather.

Cardiac rehab started early that summer just after I turned fourteen. It was an hour long, three times a week for six weeks. That was the recommended time for rebuilding my strength and reconditioning my muscles. The fellow group members were much older than I expected, and I quickly realized that I was the youngest participant. I really didn't know what to expect from rehab. It wasn't something that I chose to do. Instead, it was a prescription from the doctors that I didn't have the option of not filling.

The doctors running the sessions told us they had never had someone my age in cardiac rehab before. In that respect I felt special. Because I was younger, I received a lot of attention from my rehab comrades. They would ask me what such a young girl was doing needing this kind of rehab and would look out for me while we did our rotations on the gym equipment.

Before each session of began, I needed to put on a Holter monitor. Woohoo! They haunted me everywhere I went! These were not so terrible, with only four leads to attach. Each member had to wear a Holter, and they were linked to the computers at the desk where the nurses and doctors sat and monitored every patient's heart. My blood sugar was also checked for a baseline reading, another required precautionary measure. I didn't have diabetes. A couple of times I was encouraged to drink some orange juice before I started due to a lower than average blood sugar read. The last thing I did before our five minute warm-ups was to get on the scale. We had large, cream-colored index cards to fill out to keep track of our weight and blood pressure. Any changes were noted, the doctors called, and our fitness levels adjusted.

The rubber-band warm-ups were first. The resistance levels that you could choose from were the least resistant, yellow; to green; and then red, the most resistance. I usually went for the red while members with yellow rubber bands surrounded me, understandably so. The average ages were in their mid- to- late seventies. A few members were in their early fifties, and then there was me. The others were in rehab because of heart attacks, coronary artery disease, coronary bypasses, angioplasties, valve replacement or other cardiothoracic issues that were at the cause of their stints in rehab.

Many people were taken aback at having a young person with heart problems needing cardiac therapy. They asked a lot of questions about why I was there. "Did you have a heart attack?" "No, no heart attack," I'd reply with a smile as the group assembled to get on with the first twenty minutes of our, "workouts." I was only a little talkative about what had happened during the past few months.

I just didn't feel like sharing everything. I was still trying get over being so self-conscious about the scar. Talking about it just reminded me how bad I felt about it. A few participants told me, "This place is for old people with bad hearts." I just smiled. It was the only thing I could do to keep from answering back. I wanted to be polite and not just abruptly say, "I need to get back to my treadmill." There were several people looking out for me during my time there. All the negative feelings I had from the scar and the pacemaker started to slowly fade, and I was having fun. I was looking forward to going to my three days a week at cardiac rehab to see the nurses and the other members.

I had been Dr. Cole's and Dr. Weigel's patient for over fourteen years, and they were like family to me. We had been through a lot together. Dr. Weigel always said, "If there is anything you need, don't hesitate to call." There were nights we called the answering service to page him, and he always called us back immediately. As soon as my mom answered the phone and I found out it was Dr. Weigel, I would race to pick up the line. The three of us would chit-chat, exchanging, "How's your family doing?" and, "How is school going?" He then would get down to business and ask how I was feeling and what was going on that we needed to page him for at seven or eight at night. He was so patient, and he always answered any question, as trivial as it might seem. If he was concerned enough about what was going on, he would make sure that I got an appointment to see him as soon as possible.

During one regular check-up, Dr. Weigel left the room to go get some test results and closed the door behind him. I never could stand the door being closed and would open it so I could see everything going on in the hallway and watch as patients and the doctors passed by. It had been busy in the office that day, and mom got up to close the door. I asked if she could leave it open just a little, so she left it just about an inch open, just enough to hear the rustling squeaking of footsteps in the hallway. On the back of the door was an event flyer for the very first Children's Heart Foundation fundraiser. Mom's eyes got wide and a big grin spread across her face. She was instantly excited to learn more about how she could get involved.

Dr. Weigel wasn't two steps back in the room before she started asking about the Children's Heart Foundation. "Oh yeah, I am on the board of doctors for the foundation. You know a lot of the doctors on the board!" He said he had been working closely with the founder, Betsy Peterson and would give mom her contact information. If Dr. Weigel was involved, then it had to be something important and we would want to be involved too.

Later that night, Mom called Betsy. She was even more excited after she got off the phone. She had set up a time for us to meet with Betsy about how we could get involved. Betsy had started the foundation in memory of her son Sam, who died in 1995, when he suffered a heart-related collapse that put him into multiple organ failure. Sam was born with complex heart defects (congenital heart disease) and lived until he was eight years old. Now his memory and legacy lives on in The Children's Heart Foundation.

Mom and Betsy became instant friends. Mom became a member of the board of directors, and we began volunteering for CHF. The first fundraising event was at Chicago's Navy Pier Water Works. We took the escalator up three levels to meet up with more families, each of whom had at least one child diagnosed with a congenital heart defect. I was excited, so I rushed ahead and turned the corner to see Betsy and Dr. Weigel standing at the entrance, and then I waited for Amy and Mom to catch up. We gave Betsy and Dr. Weigel hugs, asked if Dr. Cole was coming, and inquired about the other doctors who were going to be there. Then we went on our way to explore the event. In the back of my head I was still unsure how being around other kids like me would feel. Would I get along with them? How much was I really going to share with them? I stuck close to my mom and sister. I felt comfortable with them and with Betsy, Dr. Weigel and Dr. Cole, of course. When it came to talking with the other kids, I was reluctant to share anything about myself.

The competitive side in me came out when it was time to bid on the items in the silent auction. I have always been a huge Chicago Bulls fan and only wanted the signed wooden Bulls head plaque. Michael Jordan, Scottie Pippen and Dennis Rodman were part of the greatest Bulls team in the history of the franchise and to have their three autographs together was truly exciting.

I was a huge Michael Jordan fan and had been a collector of his books and the Sports Illustrated magazines in which he was featured. He led the Bulls to a three-time, back-to-back, championship, with the last one in 1993. I watched every game and called shots as they played. Mom used to tell me I should be a sportscaster because I was good at calling the shots and yelling at the players. I was drawn to that signed Bulls head and there was little chance that I was going to lose that auction item. I still have it and it is in as perfect condition as the night I won it at the CHF fundraiser. It doesn't remind me of the Bulls, though, as much as it does the beginning of our relationship with Betsy and all the families that were a part of the foundation.

Our volunteer duties included putting together mailings for upcoming events. We were a group of about ten volunteers, made up mostly of board members. It was always a party! When we got closer to the next big fundraiser, we'd do all the stuffing, addressing and stamping of hundreds of envelopes for potential participants and donors. One board member, in particular, would host the mailing parties. She put on magnificent food spreads. There were huge bowls of chicken salad, pasta salad, fresh fruit salads, and trays of cookies, brownies and chocolates.

Our volunteer work also included the CHF annual fundraisers for the next two years. The Museum of Science and Industry hosted, and it was by far the best. Before going and enjoying the food, we had free access to the entire museum and could go explore all the exhibits.

For my volunteer job, I was stationed at the front door at a long table with five other people. I had the job of checking in the guests as they entered, and it was so entertaining. I liked talking to everyone who came through the doors. By this time, I was more open to talking with fellow heart kids who attended. I had seen some of the same families over the last few years and we had become friends.

I always had to find Dr. Cole and Dr. Weigel to exchange hugs and say hello. One year, their office staff came: Mickey, the receptionist and Laura who did all the EKGs for the doctors. It felt as if I never saw them but in reality I had either just been in the office or was coming in the following week. Dr. Weigel had mentioned that Dr. Mavroudis, the surgeon who had done my last surgery with the pacemaker, was there and that he would love to see me.

After I was done being social, Amy and I ran around the museum to see what new exhibits they had on display. We left mom to talk to the other parents she had come to know well. Mary Ann Johnson and her son Adam became good friends with the three of us. Mary Ann had been on the CHF parents' board with my mom. They shared stories and similar heart events with each other and hit it off as friends straightaway.

The Children's Heart Foundation opened up many doors for us in so many ways. It gave me connection and knowing there were other kids like me and with whom I could truly relate. It gave my sister Amy a chance to talk with other siblings and Mom a break every now and again when she attended the monthly meetings.

There weren't many well-established communities for families at that time to connect with others who were dealing with a loved one diagnosed with a congenital heart defect. Until CHF, there had been no place to share stories, compare notes on symptoms or surgeries, and just be able to talk to someone who understood the ups and downs that happened every day. In the community that we had with CHF, there were no explanations necessary for why your kid might be squatting to catch their breath or why they had a massive scar running down their chest. We had found a home and a community with this foundation.

Dr. Mavroudis told my mom after the fourth surgery that he wasn't sure he was able to do anything that actually would help. It was true. I wasn't any better after that surgery, it gave me a little more time but my heart was growing weaker. Mom figures that I had been sick, really sick since I was twelve years old. Intertwined with everything else, my migraines became worse and now were happening all the time. When I had them, the light would blind both eyes, my hearing would be super sensitive, and my head would pound even harder when I was throwing up. I would yell at my mom and say she was talking too loud when she was only whispering. I would end up lying on my bedroom floor with the room as dark as possible, curled up in a ball, and be in immense pain. The slightest movement sent pain shooting in every direction, thumping as it spread. It felt like there was so much pressure wanting to get out, just like a teakettle bursts into whistling when the steam reaches the top. The disruption in my vision was the worst, and I couldn't handle it. I would close my eyes to see if the light auras would go away, but even with my eyes closed I could see them whirling around.

We had gotten our dog Otis just after my third surgery in the winter of 1996. Amy and I had been begging mom for a dog for a while. Our previous dog Samson had passed away a year or two earlier. Since that time, I was in and out of the hospital.

We adopted Otis as a puppy. He was really sick, nearly dying due to a severe case of kennel cough and a bout of intestinal worms. As we nursed him back to health, Amy would clean his nose of dried snot and I would clear his eyes of goop. The many days I was home sick from school, he would cuddle up next to my bed and wouldn't leave my side until someone got home. He innately knew that I wasn't well, and he kept close. What was most interesting is during my migraines while I was lying on the floor, Otis would slowly walk over to see why I was crying. A few times, early on he would come up and sniff my head. We thought nothing of it at first.

Mom was always trying to find the one spot that she could press on my head to alleviate some of the pain and pressure. When Otis came in, he would nudge a little spot, always at a different place on my head, and then leave. It was as if he was trying to tell us something. Mom eventually tried applying pressure to whichever spot Otis had chosen. Sure enough, it was the right spot, the one that would take some of the pressure off so I could take a breath and have a break from the pain. Mom would press so hard on my head it hurt her hands. For me it was never hard enough. Unlike most doctors, Dr. Otis was correct every time, and his nose proved it.

The migraines just continued to get uncontrollably worse. They were so bad that I was in and out of the emergency room on a weekly basis. I saw the same ER doctor on multiple occasions, and he began to wonder if I was a morphine addict. Granted, there are people who abuse the ER to get their fix for pain medication. However, this wasn't for the morphine. I was throwing up multiple times, sometimes nearly on the doctor, and I felt like I was dying. They discontinued morphine soon after that and used Dilaudid. It was a much stronger narcotic. My pain was so bad that I had no choice. It never failed that the medication managed to mask the pain, and I got even sicker from the medication. From so many visits to the ER I become an expert at what each medication was used for, and I knew what to ask for that actually worked.

I also became an expert at asking a lot of questions when I didn't know exactly what was going on. I learned more that way than if I hadn't questioned anything the doctors told me. Perhaps, the most important lesson I learned was to never be afraid to question the doctors. They are the people who are there to answer the uncertain questions and concerns you have about your health care.

The headaches were irrepressible for nearly three days at a time and the lingering side effects had a tendency to last a few days longer. At times, my mom didn't even want to take me to the ER because of the doctors. We would drive around to see if the fresh air would help with the symptoms, but it never did. We stopped at a local restaurant for some tea one summer night in hopes that we could avoid the emergency room. I sipped my lemon and honey tea and tried to keep myself from throwing up in the restaurant. It didn't really work. The problem was nothing but a visit to the ER and the strong pain medication worked, and that was an imperfect solution.

I had multiple appointments with neurologists to rule out blood clots and brain tumors and any other brain abnormalities that might be the cause. All it proved was that I did have a brain that fit nicely within my skull. By the end, my mom had taken me to every reputable neurologist and clinic in Chicago. I was put on several different kinds of medication in hopes of controlling the migraines, but none of them worked effectively and reliably.

The last resort was a clinic renowned for the successful treatment and advances in migraine control. Only, they never figured out what was causing mine. They told me that I should do a food elimination diet, and I thought that was crazy, partly because I didn't want to do it and partly because I was barely eating much of anything, anyway. The worst part about them was they really didn't know what the hell they were doing in my case. All patients were assumed to be the same and were treated as such, and I think they had no idea how to manage such a complex case as mine. They had a good reputation and had helped many patients successfully control their migraines, but for us it was a waste of precious time.

I was worn out from going to all these doctors that gave me medication that had terrible side effects for me. Not only were my migraines kicking my ass, my heart was weakening. I was really feeling the effects of it, and they were so bad that mom had to leave CHF as a board member. The second she would leave for a meeting, I would have to call her to rush back home. She only went to meetings once or twice a month, but that was even too much. At least she could tell Dr. Weigel what was going on since he was at some of the meetings and knew when I called to have mom come home. To top the year off, my grandpa was beginning to get sick and it would be something from which he would never recover.

CHAPTER 8

Just One Day

*"How would it feel if every dream came real
And all the scars you have fade away for just one day"*
—**Better than Ezra**

Midsummer 1995, the year before my revised Fontan and pacemaker, I ended up spending two days in the hospital. I didn't quite recover from the near collapse at school earlier that year, and now my grandfather's health was becoming a serious issue. We waited for Papa to drive up to the front of the hospital, where there was a wide underpass driveway. The valets were there pulling cars in and out, as well as ambulances waiting to be called around the corner to the emergency entrance.

Looking back at this point, mom would often say, "I don't know how we did it all. If it weren't for Grandma, Papa and Annie, I don't know what we would have done." I can't even imagine how my mom did it. I was sick, she had two kids to take care of and now her father was getting sick.

Papa loved driving. A few years before he was having trouble driving, he had bought his dream sports car. It was a cherry red, two-door Dodge Stealth. He also loved his independence. The day he picked my mom and me up from the hospital was the beginning of the end for him.

He was driving us home and took the Interstate, one of the busiest three-lane highways in and out of Chicago. If you do not go fast enough, well, you are in trouble! Papa was driving in the middle lane, barely going forty-five. People were honking at him, passing him and yelling through their closed windows for him to get off the road. I was oblivious to what was going on. All I could see was Mom grasping the door handle and the console that sat between her and my grandfather. Later, she told me how scared she was that we were going to be a part of a bad accident and that someone might be killed.

When my mom was a high-school student, she worked at my grandfather's private physical therapy practice. She tended the front desk and assisted him with some of his patients. She learned very quickly how to work in a wide range of conditions. It wasn't surprising that she had begun to notice that Papa was showing very early signs of Parkinson's disease. His symptoms made sense; the tremors in his hands, lack of balance when he walked, constant falling, loss of fine motor skills and coordination, his confusion and memory loss.

Parkinson's is a progressive disorder of the nervous system that directly affects the brain. Brain cells that produce a chemical called dopamine are destroyed without being replaced by new cells. When these cells are destroyed, the patient begins to lose muscle function. It starts with tremors in the hands and gets increasingly worse as time goes on. My mom knew how devastating a disease it was, especially considering there was no cure. It was particularly trying because this was her father, a man who had been a physical therapist who helped people for a living and an active and very independent individual. This was when my mom mourned for her father the most. It was just devastating to our family. We were all so close, and the thought of Papa, a strong and unwavering man, suffering with this just killed us all. He was only sixty-nine years old and had so much life left in him.

The realization that things were about to change significantly for her father hit Mom really hard. It wasn't going to be Grandma and Papa helping us out the same way they had been able to up to now. Instead, Papa was going to need all of my grandma's attention and help, and my mom knew that. She cried, knowing her father wasn't going to get better and was going to lose his independence. She also knew what Parkinson's did to a person. She had seen it in some of my grandfather's patients when she was working for him.

Soon after that car ride home from the hospital, my grandpa's car keys were taken away. It surprised us all how easily he gave up the car. He handed them, along with his independence, over to us. We all sensed that he was relieved that he didn't have to drive anymore and that someone else had made the decision for him.

Although I wasn't in great physical shape to help with the more physically demanding tasks that grandma needed me for, we still tried to take care of Papa the best we could when we were over at their house. Amy and I helped feed him, made sure he didn't fall when he walked around the house and helped him get dressed when he needed. One day in particular, he decided he wanted his hair cut. My grandma could not take him to his usual barber because he was too unstable on his feet to walk even a short distance. If he were to fall, there was no way she could get him up off the ground. Instead, I asked Papa if he wanted me to cut his hair. "Yes, okay," he replied. I am certain he really didn't know he was saying yes to me and not to a professional. I was only fifteen and the last time I cut my hair, my bangs looked like someone cut them with their eyes closed, all uneven. Right! I actually did that, closed my eyes and cut my hair and I never did that again.

We set up a lawn chair in the back yard and sat him down. I draped a towel around him like the stylists did when they threw over the smock before starting to cut your hair. I had a small misting bottle that I used to wet the hair down and then proceeded to cut Papa's hair. I started to cut around his ears first. My hand glided neatly around one ear and the cut actually didn't look that bad. The other side did not turn out the same. I didn't have the same momentum as on the first ear. It was uneven and choppy; in fact the whole haircut turned out uneven and choppy. Usually, if something wasn't done the way my grandpa liked he would have no problem letting you know. I kept looking up at my grandma as I was cutting his hair and she just looked back and smiled, occasionally shrugging her shoulders as if to say, "Keep going, it's okay." There wasn't much more I could cut without ending up giving him a buzz cut. My grandpa was happy with it. He had no idea what a terrible job I did, but he didn't really mind the way it looked. My grandma said, "He loved that you cut his hair. You did a good job."

Papa also liked when Amy and I would tend to his nails and would often ask for us to give him manicures. I would clear off the kitchen table and Amy would get a towel and a bowl of soapy, hot water. We had a file, nail clippers, paper towels and clear nail polish ready. Amy and I took turns filing and clipping his fingernails. Grandma sat in the kitchen watching. As we would finish filing his nails, moving his hand to the soapy bowl of water, Grandma would laugh at the fact that he let us do whatever we wanted to him. Papa very much enjoyed the pampering and we had a lot of fun and liked his spa time with us. After we finished with the clear polish, we told him not to move for a while to allow the nail polish to dry. Papa would often tell us, "Go get my wallet," and he would pay us. Sometimes it was $10. That was a lot of money to Amy and me. Our mouths would drop and our eyes would widen in excitement. We never cut his hair or painted his nails to get paid. We loved that he let us do it, and that was enough. Grandma would yell at him, "That's too much money." He would brush her off and make us put the cash in our pocket so we wouldn't lose it, then he would laugh.

We used to say that Papa had healing hands. One day, I was dropped off at my grandparents' house when I had a horrible migraine that had been going for hours. At that time, Papa's tremors had gotten worse. His hands were shaking more rapidly and he was falling often. I was stalled at the front of the house because the pain had shot across my skull, stopping me in my path. Grandma had alerted Papa that Amy and I were there by yelling down the hall to him, as she often did. He came shuffling down the hallway, his pants swishing along, to see what was going on. I must have been complaining or yelling to my grandma that my head hurt. He told me, "Give me your hands," and held out his hands waiting for mine. I squinted, trying to see where his hands were, and then quickly shutting them after a piercing shot of pain rushed through the left side of my head. We both were stopped at the end of the hallway, just standing there.

My hands were on top of his hands and he began to put pressure on the thenar eminence, the group of muscles that are in the hand at the base of the thumb. Papa started pinching the muscles between my thumb and index finger first, then throughout both hands, at the same time. The second he started to apply pressure to my hands, some of my migraine pain began to dull. He had the most magical, healing hands. Next, he pressed on the bridge of my nose to alleviate some of the pressure I was feeling in my sinuses. Immediately following that, I felt much better than I had when I first got to their house. Very few people I know have a touch like that, and it's an instant healing quality that only Amy and my grandpa share. Great hands are one quality a guy must possess and thus, would explain my pickiness for hands: the right hands the right guy. But I digress; relationships are a whole other book that I will leave to the experts, like Amy Laurent, to write about.

As Papa continued to squeeze the pressure points on my hands, I closed my eyes and couldn't help but remember him in a healthy, active state. He had played handball, his sport of choice, multiple times a week. The days that I was home sick from school and long before Papa's car keys were taken from him, he and grandma would take me on spontaneous short road trips. We wouldn't go far, maybe just across the Illinois-Wisconsin border. It was just about an hour or so from their house north to Wisconsin. They might pick me up from my house and take me to lunch or to go shopping.

I know what you are thinking. Why, if I was home from school sick, would I be going out to lunch and shopping? It was the only way anyone could get me out of the house for a while. If someone didn't press me to get up and move around a little, I would have slept all day. My excessive loss of energy and constant tiredness wore me out. It was hard on my mom on those days when I couldn't go to school where teachers and the nurse could keep an eye on me. My grandparents provided her some relief from that worry. She was able to go to work knowing that I would be okay until she could get home.

There was one day in particular that stands out in my memory. I was home sick from school again, and my grandparents picked me up just after lunchtime. Papa wanted to take me strawberry picking in Wisconsin. He loved Wisconsin (He had finished a year of post-graduate work at the University of Wisconsin in Madison and was a true Badgers fan). When Papa said we were going to do something, we did it. So we went strawberry picking at a farm in Kenosha, about a half-hour past the Illinois-Wisconsin border. We walked and covered only a small part of the vast strawberry fields. It was a warm, sunny day, and I was in shorts, a t-shirt, white socks and white shoes. Papa was off filling his pint size, plastic green mesh basket with strawberries. Grandma and I tried to fill our basket with the biggest strawberries we could find. By the time we were ready to leave my white socks had become a blush of pink and red. I leaned up against the car, staring at the bright pink socks that also happened to be soaked through with water and juice from the strawberries. Grandma insisted that I take them off, and on the way home we stopped at the outlet mall and bought two new bags of white socks. Every so often in the summertime, I stop and stand in the beaming sun, take a deep breath of the fresh dewy air, and bring myself back to the strawberry fields. I can picture my grandfather in the distance picking strawberries as I lean up against their car and smile.

CHAPTER 9

Show Me What I'm Looking For

"Save me, I'm lost Oh, Lord
I've been waiting for you I'll pay any cost
Save me from being confused show me what I'm looking for."
—Carolina Liar

T he first year of high school is the beginning of the most important four years of a young person's life. It's the time when you are building lasting friendships, studying your butt off for class (well, you are supposed to be studying) and taking those ridiculous standardized tests so you can make it into college. Silly junior high crushes became high school relationship reality. Dating and hanging out with different groups of friends takes up the majority of your time, after sports and clubs are finished for the school day. It was the typical, normal stuff everyone did when entering high school. Everyone tries to find where they fit in and what activities they want to pursue during the four years of high school. For me, freshman year was hit or miss, with most of the school year being a miss. I was either out sick or barely making it through the

47

day. It was difficult for me to concentrate and really focus in class. I was often out of breath and had a hard time keeping my eyes open. All I wanted to do was sleep. My entire body was starting to give out.

Nearing the middle of the year, I could no longer make it through the whole day without the school having to call my mom at work to come pick me up. It happened so frequently that eventually Mom and the school arranged my class schedule to allow me to go home around noon every day by cab. Some days I barely made it into the house, feeling like I was going to pass out. Occasionally, I had enough energy to make myself a bowl of soup, or some noodles if I really felt up to it, which I barely ate.

In time, my high school reality was that of being taught by tutors. They came mostly after school, and it sucked. I would rather have been in school. The teachers typically came to my house around three-thirty in the afternoon. Classes were the same as if I were in school. I had Geometry, English, History and Horticulture. I was lucky to get a couple of great teachers to tutor me. Dr. P taught my history lessons and Mr. Armstrong got me through geometry. Mr. Armstrong reminded me a lot of my grandpa. I would watch out the window for him to pull up in the driveway. Every Tuesday, he walked up the sidewalk to the front door, carrying his brown briefcase. I liked when he came to tutor me because he would make me laugh, ask me how I was feeling, and then start pulling out a stack of math worksheets and our conversation would slowly move into working out geometry problems. I would look at him with a disappointed face and he would smile and say, "Time to get to work!"

I was not involved in any activities or clubs, and all I wanted to do was be in school and be a part of everything. I sometimes wonder what it would have been like if I had been able to attend high school like any other, normal student. I know for sure I would have been social and an active member of a variety of clubs. I may even have been on one of the sports teams. Tennis or golf was not completely out of the question for me to participate in. I had already missed a lot of junior high and was now looking to miss at least another year in high school.

I was fortunate to have friends who would often come visit me at home, especially Paula, after they finished school. I always wanted to see them, though I never had the energy to hang out for very long. Restless, weak, tired, drained, and struggling at times, to catch my breath was a constant feeling. When it came to having to study or focus on schoolwork, I didn't last more than ten minutes. There was never really any point where I got used to feeling like that; I just knew how to deal with it by then. My mom, on the other hand, had a harder time dealing with it because there was very little she could do to help make me feel any better. She and Amy would occasionally go to the mall to shop or pick up some food. They needed to get out of the house every now and then, too. They would run into friends of mine, healthy friends who were at the mall shopping like normal high school kids. It was hard for my mom, seeing all of them living their lives and having fun because she knew I was home, getting sicker every day. She would tell me, "Oh, I saw Heather at the mall, and she said to say hi." I would just look at her and smile. There wasn't really anything I could say. I wish I would have been there to say, "Hi!" myself, but I wasn't, and that is what, I think, hurt Mom more than it did me.

Year one of high school was done. That summer I turned fifteen and I couldn't wait to drive. I had wanted to drive since I was two years old. There was proof too, my parents had a picture of me in the driver's seat of their car when I was around three years old. I begged my mom and grandma for private driving lessons at a driving school two blocks from our house. I don't know how I made it to class every day for five weeks, I was so sick. I walked to driving school and back home. I didn't care how badly I felt, I wanted that driving permit that summer so I could practice. Otherwise, I would have to wait and take a class in school. The second I got my permit, I was in the car practicing driving in the high school parking lot. Mom and, sometimes, Amy would be in the car with me as I drove in circles around the lot and learned how to pull in and out of spaces. It was even better when mom let me drive on the street! For her, it was frightening. She would have both hands firmly holding on to the door, scared that I would hit something or jerk the car when I was trying to stop or accelerate too fast when the light changed. But, I was a really good driver, even though I had to wait until I was seventeen to actually get my license.

In Dr. Weigel's office, there was a basket of multi-flavored safety pops that sat on the right corner of the counter. It was always overflowing with candy. Every time I went in, I scoured the small basket for a purple safety pop. I was particular about the flavor I wanted: no purple grape, no pop! Amy would look for an orange one, but she was more open to having another flavor. It was the best part of the visit. When I returned for a visit, several years after my transplant, Dr. Weigel in October 2011, I found that the office no longer provides that sugary deliciousness. Believe me, I checked! He told me they got that candy from a friend who had since stopped supplying them to the office. It was a sad day for me!

On this typical high-school-day check-up, Dr. Weigel asked me how I was feeling. I explained that I was tired and sleeping a lot of the time, and that I just didn't feel good at all. Amy was now thirteen, and I had just turned sixteen. This appointment was eerily different. Dr. Weigel didn't come into the exam room with his stethoscope ready to listen to my heart. In fact, he didn't come into the room ready to do very much at all. He had been talking to Mom in the office hallway, about ten steps from the first exam room where I was. They spoke quietly at the bottom of the three short steps that led up to his office. I just sat in the room waiting for someone to come back. Mom walked in and sat down and we chatted briefly about what we were going to do after the appointment. We decided that we would get some dinner after we picked Amy up from school. A few minutes later, Dr. Weigel opened the door. He didn't have his usual smile and happy demeanor. He was, instead, quite somber.

He looked at Mom first. It was almost as if he was trying to compose himself to prepare for what he was about to say to me. Mom sat on the stool and Dr. Weigel sat down on the examining table next to me. I felt a little twinge in my stomach. I knew something was wrong. There is never a good way to tell someone bad news, but Dr. Weigel did his best. He told me that my heart was too far into congestive heart failure for them to do anything. There was nothing more they could do to repair it. The next thing out of his mouth was a curve ball that hit me square in the face he said "You need a heart transplant."

I was stunned, frozen, and all I could do was well up with tears. For at least five minutes, I sat there with tears rolling down my face. When I was finally able to produce some cohesive words, I said, "No, I don't want one." Mom came back, solemnly saying, "This is the only option." Dr. Weigel explained the details of a transplant but I didn't hear what he was saying. My ears deafened at the words "heart transplant." The only question I could barely manage to spit out was, "Will I still be able to come to you for my appointments?"

Dr. Weigel called us a few days later to see how the news was settling in. I grabbed for the phone like I did every time he called. There was more news that I didn't take very well. He said, "No, I can't be your cardiologist from now on." He would be there with me through the process, but only as a consultant because the transplant doctors needed to take over. He further explained that his specialty was solely with children. There were few adults with congenital heart problems who were still his patients. He wasn't trained to see patients with transplants. It was a whole other level of care that I needed now. Those damn curve balls kept coming at me. I guess it made sense, I just wasn't happy…at all. It felt like someone had died, like we had just lost a family member. I looked over at my mom to see if this was all really happening, and, sure enough, it was. She could only pull me in and hug me and tell me, "It will be okay," like she did so many times before. Change for anyone is difficult, and I always had a particularly hard time with it. I had always been scared of it and this change terrified me.

As we proceeded with the transplant process, we first needed to talk to the new group of doctors who would be taking me on as a new patient. Dr. Weigel thought it would be best if we went to a transplant center out of state. His top two choices were Boston Children's Hospital or Stanford University School of Medicine, near San Francisco. He felt that I wouldn't get the care and support I needed in Chicago. At the time, he couldn't change my mind: I wanted to stay in Chicago. Making that decision was the one thing I had a say in and some control over. I was stubborn and refused to go anywhere else. Ultimately, my mom would have taken me anywhere if she thought it would be for the best, but the decision to stay in Chicago was quickly made.

During that same October 2011 visit, I found out why Dr. Weigel recommended going out of state. The transplant team at the Children's hospital in Chicago took was an all-business approach. Dr. Weigel was very patient-centered, and the transplant team's approach clashed with his. Their attitude toward care and general practices were focused on getting the job done and thinking of the patient came last in many ways. This was not what Dr. Weigel thought, when he told me during my interview of him, on how the transplant team should have been practicing. Especially, when it came to working with children practically on the brink of death. I later found out just how right Dr. Weigel was when he told us that we should have gone out of state for care. The reception I received as a patient was pretty chilly. And I was just sixteen years old.

When you are in need of a lifesaving transplant, you are at the point where you have no other options. That should be pretty obvious. The only other option would have been to refuse treatment. That option never crossed my mind. I was used to fighting through illness. What was a little more fighting? I was so pissed off that I even had to have this transplant in the first place. That was the fight that kept me going. This new battle had barely just begun, and I didn't see any other choice but to move forward. The picture of me being healthy, returning to school, and being able to get back to as normal a life as possible kept me motivated. I just wanted to go back to school. I know most high school kids and probably a lot of my friends at the time would ask, "Why would you want to be in school? We wish we didn't have to go." "High school sucks, I hate the homework, teachers, gym," and so on. But, when you are not a part of something, all you want to be is a part of it.

Years later, I found out my mom was aware that before the appointment, a heart transplant was a possibility. No one knew exactly when or if it would ever become a reality. It wasn't something that we focused on. Each hypoplastic left heart syndrome (HLHS) patient is so different that there is no way of knowing whether they will ever need a new heart. Some people born with HLHS become adults and live without ever needing a heart transplant. I think my mom had a feeling early on that I was going to get to this critical point of needing a transplant.

For me, I had no idea that I could be facing a heart transplant. I was just sixteen. I was too young to either worry about it or understand all of the details and ramifications. I had always done what the doctors told me to. I never thought that needing a heart transplant was my fault, that for some reason, I hadn't done something the doctors told me to and that was the cause for a transplant. It happened that way, and there wasn't one thing I did or didn't do that caused it.

By the time I found out I was in congestive heart failure with the only cure being a transplant, shock didn't even begin to describe what was going through my head. This happened all within a matter of days when Dr. Weigel asked me if it was okay if we started the transplant process. He was going to call the hospital and get me an appointment with the transplant team as soon as possible. That was one of the last times I was under his care as his patient. There were so many milestones in my life that I shared with Dr. Cole and Dr. Weigel.

I was always excited to go visit them, even when I didn't have a scheduled appointment. They always welcomed me with open arms and big hugs. My experience after I left their practice was anything but good, supportive, or caring. My door was closing on the first 16 years of my life and just beginning to open up revealing a heart transplant and new doctors.

When you are in need of any type of organ transplant, you go through an intense workup to make sure that you are an eligible candidate to be listed and then transplanted. It was towards the middle of August, 1999, when we began. Everything needed to be done relatively quickly so I could get listed for the heart. There was a quicker way to get through everything: be admitted to the hospital. Only in dire circumstances are you admitted to be listed for a transplant, and I wasn't far from that route.

The reason patients are admitted to the hospital to wait for a transplant is it is a potentially shorter wait time if you are already in the hospital. You are more likely to be closer to the top of the list. I swiftly said no to the mere mention of this idea. I wasn't going to wait in the hospital. At that point I would have lost every bit of independence and freedom I had left. Even though I couldn't do very much, at least I could go to the bathroom without ringing a bell and waiting for a nurse to come help me.

Within a couple of weeks we had begun the first steps. I met my new cardiologist, Dr. P and her team. Dr. Weigel did everything he could to make the transition as smooth as possible for us. The process began and we met with the transplant cardiologist, cardiovascular surgeon(s), transplant coordinator, social worker, dietitian and psychologist.

In the beginning it was fine. I had no problems with my new team of doctors. I was really sick and had the mentality to do what I needed to do to get through the current situation. The one hitch and the worst part of this process were the social worker and the psychologist. I cannot express how cold, rude and completely lacking in compassion they were throughout. It is incomprehensible to me why they chose a profession dealing with children when they acted as if they didn't care what happened to the patient. They knew they had the power to say, "No, the patient isn't going to comply with the regimen the transplant aftercare requires and therefore we see they are unfit for transplant." The feeling I got from the psychologist was she hated her job and took it out on everyone. She was terrible. Dr. Weigel had to step in and explain to her that I had always been a patient who was active in her own care, took all her medications and did what the doctors asked her to do. I tried to remember it was only a step in the process that needed to get done, and I didn't want anything holding me up from being listed as soon as possible. I wasn't at all happy with the treatment and my mom let them know her opinion on the matter, too. We just tried our best to deal with it all.

Dr. P was going to take over care during and after the transplant. The other doctors involved were just there as stepping stones toward the end goal. The social worker needed to make sure I was going to be good about taking my medications. At that time I liked my new transplant doctor, Dr. P, and the transplant coordinator, Carrie.

Now for the nurse who thought she was the "social worker." Her name was Kat. She was an instigator who had no respect for me or my family. She was especially rude to my mom. She was one of the nurse practitioners who would be following me after the transplant. She did not understand nor deal with children on their level, so I didn't get why the hell she was working in a children's hospital.

I understand that the transplant teams wouldn't want to give an organ to patients who are not likely to not keep up with his or her medication regimen. You could suddenly feel great, think you are cured, and then stop taking the medicine. I got why they asked about my history of taking medication. I had learned to take and manage my medications from the time I was five years old. Patients who had never taken medications on a regular basis might be a concern and it is natural for the nurses and doctors to be skeptical of their habits. Of course, I had occasional mishaps where I accidentally spilled an entire bottle of pills down the sink or left all my medication at home when we went on vacation. It happened, and my parents were never happy when it did. I would hear, "Oh Jessica, not again. You can't open a full bottle of pills over the sink!" But that is what the pharmacy and your doctor were for, to call in an emergency refill. Believe me we had to go that route a couple of times. I admit I was sometimes clumsy or forgetful and opening a bottle of pills by the sink was really not a good idea! (My pill bottles now sit in my room on my desk so if I happened to spill the bottle, I can pick them up, No emergency refill is necessary). My mom told the social worker, who was also nasty and unnecessarily interrogated me, that I had always been good about taking my medicine. The social worker finally accepted that answer, passing that part of the process.

The dietician came in to ask me about my eating habits. Overall, I explained, I was a pretty healthy eater. I rarely ate fried foods and I stopped eating red meat when I was five. I rarely ate meat, and when I did, it was turkey and sometimes a little fish. I have disliked fast food since becoming a vegetarian. It wasn't for any cardiac or health reasons, it just became my preference.

By the end of August, I was finished with all the required tests and pre-qualification paperwork, and now I could officially be listed for the heart. The final meeting with Dr. P and Carrie was to inform my parents and me that I was listed and what that meant. They asked if we had any more questions for them. I just smiled and said, "Thank you." They explained that I would receive a pager within the next couple of weeks. This would allow the hospital to get hold of us when a heart became available.

The expected wait time on the list was anywhere from six to twelve months. It could potentially be longer, and you were lucky if it was shorter. Dealing with the transplant team was nothing like the experience I had had with Dr. Cole and Dr. Weigel. It was the least supportive care I had received in sixteen years, and it was hurtful. By no means am I saying that the knowledge the doctors had was bad, they were brilliant in the field, but it was their bedside manner and lack of ability to deal with someone my age that hindered the relationship. From the beginning, I had a feeling that we were not going to be happy with the future care.

CHAPTER 10

One Fine Day

"The arms I long for, will open wide
And you'll be proud to have me
Walkin' right by your side
One fine day you're gonna want me for your girl."
– Carole King

A few months before I got on the transplant list, my mom had contacted Starlight Children's Foundation to ask them to grant me a wish. Starlight is an organization that grants wishes for children diagnosed with serious, life-threatening and terminal illnesses. By that July, a woman from the organization, Marci Friedman, called my mom to say they were going to grant me a wish, and that Marci would be helping us make the best wish possible. After thinking over what I really wanted to do I told my mom that I wanted to go to New York City. My top choices had always been to meet Michael Jordan or meet the Chicago Cubs or even meet N'SYNC, which was wildly popular in

1999 and could be really fun. My mom and Marci both agreed that it should be something a bit more special and unique than just meeting professional athletes, musicians or other celebrities. Those were popular wishes. I knew I wanted it to be something that my mom and sister would enjoy with me. My mom had always talked about how she would love to take Amy and me to New York one day to see plays on Broadway. She didn't have to talk me into the idea of going to New York. It was the perfect wish. Amy and I had never been to New York, and I was getting excited just talking about it.

Marci granted my wish and made it an experience that not one of us Amy, my mom, Mom's friend Barbara, nor I would ever forget. Marci called the house nearly every day to see how we all were doing and if there was any news on the transplant front. Then she would update Mom on the reservations she had made: the plane tickets, the hotel and the Broadway show "Annie Get Your Gun" with Bernadette Peters. She asked me as much as possible about why I chose to go to New York and what I wanted to do when we were there. She used all that information to tailor the trip to my vision. She stopped by the house, bringing little gifts that we could use on the trip. She brought us a travel book of New York so we could start looking and mapping out all of the places we wanted to visit. She was amazing and put this elaborate wish together for me in only a short couple of months. She went above and beyond to make even the hardest days better. She really gave all of us, not just me, something good and exciting to look forward to.

In the meantime, we had been waiting to get the pager in the mail from the hospital. It took about two and a half weeks. I am not sure why it took so long. To add to the frustration of the wait, we missed the package the day UPS delivered it to the house. It was imperative that we pick it up the night of the missed delivery to be able to activate it the following day.

I held the small padded envelope containing the pager on my lap as we drove back home from UPS. I opened the manila envelope with the bubble wrap lining and pulled out the "doctor style" pager. I looked at it and thought, "I don't know what I am supposed to do with this," tossed it back in the envelope and flung it on the table. Is Mom going to hold on to it or am I? I didn't want it.

Our New York trip was booked for October 2, 1999. Marci called on Saturday night, it was a week before we were leaving for New York. She and Mom were discussing the itinerary she had put together for the trip. Marci had made dinner reservations for the night we arrived in New York, and Mom was going to buy tickets to the play *Chicago*. About half an hour after talking to Marci, the phone rang again. It was the hospital. Mom thought it was a little odd for the hospital to be calling after eight o'clock on a Saturday night, but she didn't think too much of it at the time. "Yes, this is Eileen, Jessica's mom," she said to the nurse. We hadn't even set up the pager yet so she initially thought that was what the call was about.

Amy and I were sitting in her room watching, of all things, a reality medical trauma show. There was a segment where a person had been in an accident and was taken into the emergency room with blood gushing everywhere. I turned to Amy and said, "Oh, that's gross!" Amy made an agreeable face back at me.

We were going to New York in exactly one week. We knew mom had been talking to Marci so we were both waiting for her to come up and tell us what she had said about the trip. What happened in the next ten minutes was a complete blur. The phone rang, it was the hospital and mom had already picked it up and was listening to the transplant coordinator Julie, explain what we needed to do. I picked up the phone and heard that it was the hospital. I started crying and yelling, screaming that I didn't want to go. Mom came running up the stairs yelling "we need to go now! We got the call for your heart".

I answered, "I'm not going anywhere."

Mom said, "You have to go, the hospital called and said they have a heart for you. Let's go, now!"

We had a short window of time to get downtown to the hospital, roughly two hours. They needed to get me checked in and prepped for surgery. It takes nearly six hours to coordinate everything for transplant. The transplant coordinator said the doctors were on their way to harvest the heart just as we were on our way to the hospital. The doctors still had to make sure the heart was viable, that it was healthy and in good condition to be transplanted. They don't know what the condition of the heart is until they physically examine it. You get the call saying you have a match blood type, size and all of the initial match requirements, and then you have to get yourself to the hospital immediately. There was always a chance you would get to the hospital and the heart wouldn't be healthy enough to procure.

Well, it was not that easy to get me out of the house. All I could think about was that we were supposed to leave for New York the next weekend. Couldn't I just wait to get the heart when we got back? What was wrong with that? After all I had only been on the transplant list for three weeks when the call came in. No one expected it to happen that fast. In the end, there is a reason for everything. Who knows how much longer I really could have lasted while waiting for a heart. I speculate that it probably wasn't much longer, and it didn't hit me until later that I got one just in time.

At that moment, I was really upset. I was so pissed off that I threw the remote on the floor. I should have been happy about getting the call, especially so soon after going on the list, but New York, New York, New York just kept bombarding my thoughts. I actually started crying over it. In the midst of all this, Amy and mom were trying to get me to leave the house. She called my father to tell him we got the call for the heart and he needed to come over to help get me into the car to leave for the hospital. I was in my pajamas running around the house crying, and I refused to get dressed.

My father made it to the house and tried talking to me, explaining that we needed to go and time was limited. Mom assured me that Marci would reschedule the trip for after the transplant. We could still go to New York, just not next weekend. My father and Amy were getting me ready to go the best they could, and Mom was finishing making phone calls to let people know we got "the call."

She had to call her friend Barbara who was to go with us on the trip that it was going to be rescheduled. Then we were headed downtown. Mom also called my grandparents, my uncle, my aunt and Mike, who she was supposed to have a first date with that Sunday.

I had made it several feet into the garage but not yet into the car. Mom and Amy said anything they could to talk me into just getting into the car. Then Amy remembered that I had wanted to go horseback riding again someday. We had been riding once before on a trail in Colorado with my father. I loved it. Amy, on the other hand, had the worst riding experience, ever! Her horse was stubborn and wouldn't move no matter what she did to try and get him to go forward. Just thinking about her face while on the horse makes me laugh. Her nose was scrunched up and she looked so upset because her horse was stalling way behind the rest of the group. The trail guide had to hold her horse's reins for the entire trail, about an hour's ride. It was a traumatic horse experience for her, and she refused to ever do it again. She was also around eight years old and instances like that could scare any eight-year-old out of doing it again.

Amy said, "I will go horseback riding with you when you feel better," and I stopped dead in my tracks. I had just made it to the door of the porch. "Just get in the car and we can talk about it on the way to the hospital." With that, I huffed my way to the car and got in. I asked Amy, "Do you promise?" Amy said, "I promise." I am still waiting to go horseback riding with her, by the way.

We were all finally on our way to the hospital. My father followed behind us, and Barbara and my uncle were going to meet us at the hospital. I asked Mom if she had talked to Grandma. She said that she couldn't get hold of her or Papa. We had no idea where they were, and they didn't have cell phones. My grandma and grandpa knew from the beginning that I was being worked up for the heart transplant, and we told them I was officially on the waiting list the minute we knew.

My uncle and my mom tried calling my grandparents again to let them know we had gotten the call for the heart and that we were all at the hospital. I tried calling the house myself at least three times to check and see if they had gotten home. Each time, Great Grandma Annie answered the phone. She told me they were not home, and she didn't know where they were or when they would be home. Several nights a week they went out to dinner and played poker with friends, rarely ever missing a game. "I don't know where they are. No they are not home yet." It was around 11:15 p.m. when I called, again. It wasn't out of the ordinary that I called often to see where they were so I don't think Annie caught on to why we had been calling the house so much. She asked me if everything was alright. At that time, I just couldn't tell her that we were at the hospital waiting for the cardiac surgeons to fly back with my new heart.

It had only been two weeks since telling Annie that I needed a new heart. When we were at my grandparent's house, my grandma, mom, sister and I would whisper about what was going on. I didn't know, if anything, what Annie knew and I hated keeping secrets from her. I decided it was time to tell her what was going on with my health. I went to her bedroom at the end of the hall, where she was watching TV as per usual. I walked over to her little couch where she was sitting, sat on her lap, and began telling her about how I was sick again and this time I was going to need a heart transplant. I felt her sink back into the couch a bit. I wrapped my arms around her and she did the same. We cried. I told her that I was going to be ok, I promised I would. She stroked my hair and rubbed my back as she always did. I told her that I loved her very much and I walked back to the living room and told my mom and grandma "Annie knows and she is ok."

Annie was home alone and all she would do was worry. I asked if she would have Grandma call one of us as soon as they got home, told her I loved her and that I would call her tomorrow. I hung up the pay phone in the family waiting room where my family was nervously waiting and I was pacing the room, until I could be moved in to a room.

My mom, Amy, Barbara, my father and my uncle, had all been in the little waiting room with me trying their best to distract me from staring out the small window in the door waiting for the nurse to appear. She could be coming in to get me at any time, I just didn't know when and the wait was driving me crazy. Then, almost magically, she was in the doorway. She motioned for me to come with her so she could get an IV started and to give me some medications before I went down to the operating room.

I was in a small room, sitting on a gurney with wheels, not a very stable place to try and start an IV. The nurse leaned up against the bed when she was trying to check for places to put the IV, and the bed would slide against the wall. That little room had carts full of hospital gowns next to the bed. To occupy my mind, I just stared at them and, occasionally, looked back at my arm where the nurse was trying to go in with the needle. I was not a patient who looked away when the IV went in. I needed to watch every step carefully to make sure she was doing it correctly. I could tell immediately when an IV would work and when it would blow and blood would erupt from the vein that just went flat and was no longer a usable access site.

This time, it took the nurse only two tries before she got the IV started. We were then off to a regular patient room where I could put my overnight bags down and "relax." I am not sure what the word "relax" means in a hospital context, nor did I ever figure that out. How can you "relax" when you are preparing to have a heart transplant in mere hours?

The heart was good. My family and I were informed that the heart the doctors viewed was healthy and they would be flying back, reaching the hospital within the hour.

CHAPTER 11

September

"Our hearts were ringing in the key our souls were singing."
—Earth Wind and Fire

E verything in a hospital is hurry up and wait…a long time. It's a typical characteristic of hospitals. The doctors seem to take their time, or take on too many patients at once, and then the patients are left waiting what seems like a ridiculously long time. Our rush to get to the hospital once we got the call for a heart turned into a three-hour wait before the doctors were ready for me in the O.R. I wasn't complaining about the wait time this time. I understood that all the doctors needed the time to be prepared. It was 1999, and though heart transplants had been being done successfully for years, they were still new and a very big deal.

None of that lessens the fact that I hate the waiting game in the hospitals. Part of it is that I can't keep myself occupied enough to distract me from why I am there.

I have learned to try and be more patient, to slow down. Otherwise I miss the bigger picture; I am not in the moment anymore. What if those moments before the surgery were my last with my family, ever? Would they remember me asking when the doctor was getting back, where the nurse was, what's going on now? I wanted to focus on spending that time not complaining and just being with the people I love and who love me the most. We still hadn't gotten hold of my grandparents.

As soon as the doctors in the operating room were ready, they called the nurse who was taking care of me. She mentioned to me earlier that night when she was trying to put the IV in for what seemed like the millionth time, "Tonight I get to see you get your new heart!" She explained that there was a place she could go, the gallery, to watch the surgery. I pictured it being like an episode of *Grey's Anatomy* or *House* where the resident doctors and nurses watch from an observation room directly above the operating room. I am sure it is not nearly as dramatic as they make it out to be on TV, but I assume the hospital had something like that. Except, there was no drama like there would be on TV. No one was arguing about who was dating whom or daydreaming of being on a white sandy beach somewhere exotic. Then suddenly, the doctor who was supposed to be focusing on surgery snaps back into reality, jolts back and oops, a major artery is cut. Blood is everywhere, and the patient is flat-lining. The doctors begin arguing, blaming each other, screaming over the patient. A nurse yells to break up the fight and all is repaired and the patient is saved. I definitely know I saw an episode of _House_ like that. I didn't think my time was going to be anything like that scenario, but the nurse might have been entertained by it! My surgeons were serious and all business, so I was confident that a scene out of one of these shows was unlikely.

I smiled and shrugged my shoulders slightly at the fact that the nurse was going to be watching my transplant. I really didn't know what to say, if she was excited, great. I just wanted to get through it already. I just didn't want to think too much about everything that was about to take place. I got the feeling that this was going to be my nurse's first time watching a heart transplant and I can appreciate why she was so excited about it. The children's hospital had only recently started performing heart transplants a few years earlier. I was the seventy-fifth patient to receive a heart at that hospital. I remember my mom telling me that after the doctors were done with my transplant, they were going right into the seventy-sixth patient late Sunday, early Monday morning, nearly twenty-four hours straight, in the operating room for the surgeons that weekend. Talk about being on your feet for a long time!

It had to be close to two o'clock on Sunday morning when the doctors were ready for me. Usually, for any test or surgery when you are an admitted patient, you are wheeled down on one of the hospital beds, called transportation gurneys, and sometimes it sucks and is embarrassing because people know you are sick. People look at you, even though the other patients have to do the same thing. It's sort of like the way people can't help but look when there is an accident on the highway. When you're the one they are looking at, there is just something about it that makes you feel so helpless. Obviously they have you on the gurneys for a reason, but sometimes it just feels like everyone is looking at you when all you want to do is run the other way. That's how I felt. Maybe I was making too much of it, but it was one more thing I did not have control over.

This time was different. The nurse asked me if I wanted to get wheeled to the operating room or walk. Of course, I chose to walk there. I hugged my Uncle Rich and Barbara who told me, "Good luck!" My mom, sister and my father walked down with me as we followed the nurse to the O.R. Sometimes people say it felt like they were moving in slow motion, when something traumatic was happening. When we were all walking down, it didn't feel like slow motion at all. In fact, it all happened relatively quickly.

I always imagined all the operating rooms were located in the basement of hospitals. It is probably because they are the "scary" places in the hospital where no one wants to go. In reality, the operating room I was headed to was on the second or third floor. The whole time we were walking, I kept shifting my hospital gown back onto my shoulder. I was pretty thin and the hospital gowns were far bigger than me and always were slipping off my shoulder. Have I complained about the gowns yet? Since they never close in the back I was wearing two, as I always did when I couldn't get away with wearing my own comfy clothes. I also had on those blue socks with the rubber bottoms. I tried to get away with wearing my own socks but my nurse made me change. She said that the socks the hospital provides are so you can walk around the hospital and not have to worry about slipping. Such a fashion statement! What if there was a gorgeous surgeon waiting for me in the O.R.? The doors would fling open and there I am, wearing a frumpy hospital gown, blue rubber socks, my hair a mess and no makeup on. That's a girls nightmare right there! I was sixteen, after all.

We got off the elevator and walked down the gray cement tiled hallway. It was quite chilly. The hospitals do that on purpose; it helps prevent more bacteria from living and spreading. Bacteria breeds and multiplies in places that are very warm. Preventing bacterial infections in the O.R. is especially important during surgery. Once you make that first incision, the risk of infection increases.

We walked through the first set of two, large steel doors. Just before the second set of swinging doors, we came to a stop. My mom, sister and my father had been following us down the hallway. The nurse turned to them and said, "This is as far as all of you can go. Take your time, and say I love you here." It was not even ten feet away from the O.R. door when we stopped. We weren't the type of family to say goodbye when it came to every surgery or test I had. We always just said we would see each other later. I tried to picture what I would be doing after this was over. This technique had helped me through a lot of situations before, and this one wasn't any different.

I was looking forward to being healthy again and everything I was going to be able to do. New York was still on the schedule, and I couldn't wait to get there. I gave mom a hug first, then Amy and then my father. I went back to my mom and gave her another hug and told her I loved her. I hugged her as tight as I could. I didn't want to let go, but I knew that I had to. I was staring my future in the face and had to get on with it.

The nurse held the door to the O.R. open. I said, "I love you," again to my family and walked in. There was no turning back now. I had one foot inside the operating room door and the O.R. nurses were already walking over to greet me. The first thing that caught my eye was the eerie, big, alien-like light that hung over the operating table. It was so bright. The operating table was slightly to my left and the doctors and nurses were running around putting the finishing touches on their preparations. A nurse guided me to the operating table where they got me settled in and relaxed. Thank goodness for that medication! The next thing I remember was waking up in my ICU room, three days later.

A couple hours before I walked into the operating room, I started my first dose of anti-rejection medications. It is common for transplant patients to get a dose before or during the transplant to prevent rejection of the organ. These immunosuppressive drugs do exactly what they sound like: suppress the immune system. It leaves the door wide open for getting very sick with infections, colds and other potentially serious illnesses that a normal person wouldn't necessarily get really sick from. Germs are a transplant patient's worst enemy and they are everywhere. If the immune system isn't suppressed immediately, the risk of immediate rejection of the heart is very possible, if not inevitable. The body sees it as a foreign object and is ready to attack and kill it. What it doesn't realize is that by doing so, it will put you back on the transplant list.

This is where those perfectly itchy and slightly suffocating surgical masks come to play. My mom happened to get a really bad cold during the three days I was out. When I woke up from the anesthesia, I wanted to see her. In she came, wearing a mask, coughing and Kleenex in hand. The doctors allowed her in my room to sit with me as long as she wore a mask. I couldn't have anything from home in my ICU room. The doctors told us they carried too many germs, even though they were my belongings with my own germs. It just wasn't going to happen. I kept pushing the doctor, asking her if I could keep one little stuffed animal in my room. My mom had just bought me a little stuffed mouse with green overalls and a flower behind her ear. Mom and Amy always got little stuffed animals to keep with me when they couldn't be there. One of my favorites was a little painted wooden heart with wings that hung on a doorknob.

My mom couldn't stay with me every night at the hospital. Even though she wanted to, she had to take care of Amy and herself in order to be able to take care of me once I was released. I couldn't risk getting sick so I understood. The doctor finally gave in, and the little mouse they bought me sat on the windowsill across from my bed, where I could see it. She put her rules down: the stuffed animals and other gifts were to stay out of my hospital bed and only be allowed on the windowsill. I could live with that.

I never had to request a private room at the hospital again. Transplant patients get their own rooms so as not to be surrounded by other patients who are sick. My room in the ICU had one window looking out to the nurse's station and the other, where my mouse sat, looking out on the busy street below. One day when I was awake enough to know what was going on, I glanced out the window to watch the autumn leaves blowing in the rainy wind. I thought how nice it would be to be outside instead of stuck in an uncomfortable, noisy bed. I was in a lot of pain and tried to get the attention of one of the nurses through the window that looked out to the nurse's station. I had no idea where the call button was and for some reason, they didn't come around much to check to see how I was doing. I didn't know it at the time, but this was just a glimpse of my future care.

My mom came in to find me in excruciating pain. I told her how I tried to get the nurse's attention and how I tried to yell, but my voice was hoarse and weak. I didn't know where my call button was and no one had come around to check on me in a while. My mom wasn't at all happy to hear that, and she left. The next thing I knew, I was watching her through the window of my room, and she wasn't happy or nice at this point at all. The nurses checked up on me quite a bit more often after that.

My whole body was swollen. I looked down at my hands because I couldn't figure out why they hurt so much and why they were barely moving. I remember asking myself why they were so big and so swollen. I had no idea how much medication was started during those three days I had been sleeping and what side effects it was having on me.

One of the after-transplant medications used to help prevent rejection is Prednisone, a wicked drug that is very effective at helping to prevent organ rejection. It is a strong steroid, and I was started at a hefty dose of 100 mg. It left my body in total disarray. Prednisone was part of my new medication regimen, and it didn't look like it was going anywhere anytime soon. All my previous medications had been replaced. Capoten (Captopril), a drug that treats congestive heart failure and high blood pressure and Furosemide (Lasix), a diuretic that treats fluid retention had been my normal regimen for years. Coumadin was added after I received the pacemaker to help thin my blood and prevent clots from forming. Throughout those years, the doctors started and stopped numerous migraine medications because nothing ever worked to prevent the onset of the headaches.

My new set of medications was totally different. I started taking Prograf (Tacrolimus) and Cyclosporine (Neoral) to prevent rejection and at least twelve other medications, like Prednisone and Bactrim to help fight infections.

I spent another two-and-a-half weeks in my own room on the transplant floor. Within those remaining weeks, I was headed to the cath lab every other day. Since risk of rejection is highest right after transplant, the multiple heart catheterizations with biopsies were necessary to check for rejection. If I was rejecting, it would be caught early enough to treat. The cath labs are just like the operating room; large white lights, small stainless steel table in the middle of the room, surgical supplies everywhere and four different computer monitors ready for viewing.

Before I went into the cath labs, my mom told me, and all the nurses and doctors, a story about when I was five years old. I was in the hospital for a cardiac catheterization just before undergoing my third heart surgery. Dr. Muster performed nearly every cath I had as a baby and toddler. He was a very serious doctor and rarely cracked a smile or laughed while doing his job. When I was old enough to comprehend, my mom would do a good job of explaining procedures and doctors' visits. This time my mom explained that the cath was going to allow the doctor to look inside my body. I am sure I answered, "Okay," as I often did. Mid-cath I woke up and asked Dr. Muster if it was Halloween. The ever-serious doctor came to the family waiting room still laughing. My mom and grandma were there and couldn't figure out why he was smiling. "She woke up in the middle of the procedure and asked if it was Halloween! I couldn't figure out why she was asking me that." My mom said it was because Halloween meant skeletons to me and I must have figured that was what the doctor was looking at my skeleton. The mind of a five year old is very imaginative, but it seemed to make sense at the time. Through the cardiac catheterizations, the doctors did find that I was in the early stages of rejection. Luckily it was at the lower end of the chart, a 2B. It meant that the heart was unstable (rejection). And that meant an increase in my Prednisone dosage, a 50-mg. increase to bring the grand total to150 mg. It was way too high, if you ask me, but I couldn't argue on this one. I needed Plasmapharesis treatments for the first few days after the transplant. My antibody levels were higher than the doctors wanted. These were markers that indicated my new heart would likely be harmed if not treated. My body would see that tissue as an invader and would want to get rid of it as fast as it could.

Human blood is comprised of red and white blood cells, platelets and plasma. The blood cells: red, white and platelets are then returned to the body with new plasma or a, "plasma like" substitute, the liquid part of the blood that doesn't contain cells. If you take plasma out, you have to replace the plasma that is removed with new plasma or a plasma substitute (acts as if it were the real thing). The autoantibodies (proteins found in the plasma) are what wrongly attack the body's new organ and those autoantibodies need to be removed and replaced.

The nurse who ran the plasma machine had to put another IV in for the treatment to begin. I needed three plasma exchange treatments and the first IV, a green butterfly needle, was placed in my groin. Four hours later, it was removed. These treatments were only given while I was in the ICU and each time I needed to sit for four hours with a new IV each time. Good thing the following IVs were in my arm. I questioned the plasma nurse about using my two other IVs and her response was, "we need a clean line so there is less of a chance of any remaining medications or fluids entering the line during the cleaning process." "Ugh, fine, whatever. Do what you have to do." You go into the OR with one IV and come out with three or four in completely random places only to be surprised that you need ANOTHER one put in. The plasma machine was massive, loud and took up all of the space there was between my bed and the door into my room. I had a hard time sleeping those hours the machine was on and now the pain of the surgery was slowly starting to show itself. It was a much different pain than I was feeling from all of the swelling.

CHAPTER 12

Calling All Angels

"I need a sign to let me know you're here.
All of these lines are being crossed over the atmosphere
I need to know that things are gonna look up
'Cause I feel us drowning in a sea spilled from a cup."
—Train

The question I get asked the most is, "Do you know who you got your heart from?" It is an added gift if you are lucky enough to know the generous family who donated their loved one's organs. We never found out who donated their child's organs so that I and seven other people could live the night we got the call. My mom had heard on the news that a local fifteen-year-old Chicago girl had been shot that night and had died of brain injuries. Her family had donated her organs and, naturally, we wondered if that was the family that had saved my life. I insist that this is only an assumption, we never really knew for sure.

Shortly after my surgery, my mom wrote a letter thanking my donor family for the selfless gift, telling them how I might not have survived without this transplant. We never got a response back, but we also understand how hard it must have been to respond to a letter thanking them for this gift in the midst of their loss. Everyone deals with loss differently, and we understood. At the beginning, I was interested in knowing my donor family, but as time went on, the desire to reach out to them waned. My mom is the one who would still like the opportunity to reach out in gratitude, but I feel that it should be left alone.

As much as my mom would have liked to be able to thank the family in person, it comes with the territory. Some families don't want to revisit the loss of a loved one. A thank you from someone who survived because of their loss might only serve to make them question again why their loved one had to die. It is emotional. No matter which side you are on, the loss is felt all around. There is no winner, only one girl who got to live. So I again say, "Thank you."

My mom had missed her date with Mike that Sunday, but he was at the hospital with her the next few days. A couple of days after the transplant, Marci came to the hospital to visit my family in the ICU. I looked out the little window my room door had in it and saw my mom and Marci outside talking. Marci was standing just outside the window and when we caught site of each other, she waved to me as she tried to balance the oversized tray of food she had special delivered for my family, making sure everyone had something to eat besides hospital food. It was a huge tray full of all kinds of sushi. Mom and Amy had to pass on the sushi because they are allergic to fish. My father and Mike ended up eating most of it, so at least someone got to enjoy it. I so badly wanted to eat some sushi right along with them as my appetite was slowly returning, and I couldn't wait to eat something. My mom finally got ahold of my grandparents and great-grandma the morning after I received the heart. They came to the hospital a few days later. I was still in and out of a fog, but I remember Papa and Annie coming in my room to see me. I was only allowed two visitors at a time.

The protective gear is so fashionable! Visitors to my room in the ICU had to wear a mask, a gown that looked like a jumpsuit and shoe covers in order to prevent any outside germs from coming in. My immune system was too weak for even my grandparents to enter the room without getting dressed up. I still have an image my great-grandma and grandpa coming in fully clothed in the jumpsuit and shoe covers. I was happy to see them, but all I could do was smile and mutter, "I love you." Grandma waited in the family waiting room, talking to my mom, while Annie and Papa visited with me for a couple of minutes.

Papa was becoming less steady. He dragged his feet more and couldn't balance himself as he shuffled about. He was becoming slower, not only physically, but mentally. When I would try to ask him questions, his answer were always the same, "Okay." The Parkinson's was beginning to be more evident. Of the three of them, Grandma was the only one who could drive. After Papa's keys were taken away, Grandma was in charge of driving him and Annie, who was ninety-three and had never learned to drive.

My mom and sister weren't required to wear masks and protective gear to that extent; I had already been exposed to their germs because we all lived together and it wasn't as much of a concern.

The rest of the time I spent in my room on the transplant floor was tough. I was in so much pain I didn't know what to do with myself. My back was killing me and I began to have really bad cycles of migraines that lasted three days at a time, easily. It was painful to lie down, sit up, or walk around. The slightest draft or touch of my bed sheets sent the pain deeper. Everyone took turns trying to massage the knots out of my back and shoulders, but the relief did not last long. The doctors didn't like to give pain medications and, as much as I pleaded for something to take a little of the pain away, they refused. They allowed me to take Tylenol every four to six hours, but that had little to no effect. I don't think the doctors truly understood the kind of pain I was in. Most of them had not experienced something like that themselves, and it was hard to make them understand how much I needed some pain relief. My migraines were bad. At that point, I don't think there was one thing that didn't hurt me.

On a positive note, my appetite was returning and mom was happy to hear I wanted to eat. That was a good indication that I was starting to feel better. Mom was willing to get me whatever I wanted. The side effects of the Prednisone were definitely present.

I had visitors, once I moved from the ICU, in and out of my room the remainder of the time I was in the hospital. My mom gave everyone daily updates on my progress. A couple of times, Betsy came to visit. During one of her visits, out of nowhere I decided I was hungry and the only thing that would satisfy this particular craving was popcorn. It wasn't just any popcorn, but the best popcorn in Chicago: Garrett's Popcorn on Michigan Avenue. Betsy and my mom giggled at my food choice and my mom had asked the nurse to make sure I was allowed to eat the popcorn before she bought it. I was restricted from eating a good number of food items until at least six months out from the transplant date. The doctor approved the popcorn, and Betsy told my mom she would take her to Garrett's to get some caramel and cheddar cheese popcorn. It was the traditional, "Chicago Mix" and my mouth waters every time I think about it. It was another tradition that Amy, mom and I made after visits to the doctor.

Betsy picked my mom up from the hospital and they left for Garrett's popcorn on Michigan Avenue which was only a few blocks away. They weren't gone more than twenty minutes when Betsy and my mom walked into my room with a large bag of Garrett's Chicago Mix. My mom tried to hold herself back from laughing as she started to say, "She made me get out in the middle of Michigan Avenue!" It is very rare that street parking along Michigan Avenue is available as it is an extremely busy street with a lot of traffic and people. With no place to park, as mom proceeded to explain, "Betsy told me to get out, in the middle of the street. She told me to go get the popcorn and that she would come back around the corner to pick me up." The line at Garrett's is consistently out the door and around the corner. It is a popular stop when you are in Chicago and the smell is too hard to resist; that buttery, fresh popped aroma that flows through the street is intoxicating. That day, when Betsy and Mom went to get popcorn, the line wasn't any shorter than out the door and around the corner. Betsy ended up driving around the block several times before Mom finally got to Garrett's, got in the door, ordered and paid. They both thought the whole experience was funny, and if you ask them about it today, they'll both start laughing and will be happy to tell you of their adventure all over again.

Yes, food! I am a total foodie, but the hospital is not the place to be sampling top food items. Most of the time, it's pretty inedible. Hospital food is an inpatient's best friend and worst enemy. I couldn't complain too much because they did have better cafeteria food than most hospitals. I always knew that when I didn't feel like eating, there was something going on. I love to eat. While I am in the middle of eating one meal I think about what I want to eat for my next meal. Unfortunately, when you are stuck in the hospital, the food is less than impressive. I think that sometimes the hospital, as much as it tries to save your life, also tries to kill you with their food offerings. The standard hospital food tray comes with the old, scratched up, blue plate covering that drips condensation on a not-so-tasty, seemingly "good for you" food. I can still smell the salty chicken broth flowing from the cafeteria. It somehow gets into every part of the hospital and it does not mix well with the smell of saline and alcohol. For me, the food is the most important part of every one of my hospital stays. My mom would tell me she knew when I felt better. I would request real food from somewhere outside the hospital, unless it was from a Starbucks or other café the hospital had on the first floor. Perhaps any patient, who has spent at least several days in the hospital, can empathize with me when it comes to eating hospital food.

When the hospital room menu came around, and I didn't have any diet restrictions, I would make it clear to the nurses that I didn't eat meat by writing on the top of the paper menu "Vegetarian!" I have been known to cry over food trays that were delivered to me completely wrong. It doesn't help when I am starving and get the wrong tray containing a hamburger or turkey sandwich. My go-to hospital order, ever since I could remember, was mini cheddar cheese squares with carrots, celery and ranch dressing. Occasionally a peanut butter and grape jelly sandwich would do the job, but only around eleven at night when I was allowed to have a snack. Mini cereal boxes were also my best friends. I used to ask for two boxes at breakfast and save them so I would have something to eat later on. There were times I wasn't able to eat in order to prepare for a test. Other times I didn't get a chance to eat due to late nights in the ER waiting to go home or to be admitted to the hospital and taken to a room. It was those times that I was so hungry and just wanted to eat something.

My mom and sister were always rushing around trying to satisfy my appetite and keep me as comfortable as they could when I was in the hospital. Amy would say, "We would get her something she wanted, and she'd take two bites and say, 'I am done.'" I do not know why food was always so important to me. Maybe it was because it gave me a focus and something to look forward to, even though most of the time I could never eat all that much without getting sick to my stomach. The early morning appointment breakfasts consisted of cereal and hash browns for me. Amy usually got oatmeal and mom always got two hard-boiled eggs, a couple strips of bacon and a small cup of grits. It's weird to remember, but I can still see the breakfast laid out, piping hot, and the cafeteria ladies knowing what to get for us. My mom always says, "It is scary when people get to know you that well at a hospital." We always had someone asking how we were all doing or, "What are you here for today?" Amy and I occasionally got frozen yogurt between or after appointments. The chocolate and vanilla swirl with Oreo crumbs was my favorite and Amy usually got strawberry flavor with rainbow sprinkles.

Food was also a big part in our routine that Mom, Amy and I had. It wasn't the food itself. It was being together in a restaurant where we just take a breath, share a laugh or some tears. Our favorite, "debriefing" spots were R.J. Grunts, best salad bar ever, followed by a walk through the Lincoln Park Zoo. Lindo Mexico was a favorite, and often visited, spot where the chips and salsa flowed freely. For the longest time, Amy refused to eat any type of ethnic food, and Mexican was no exception. After a lot of coaxing, we got Amy to try some tacos. From then on, she enjoyed the times we went to our favorite Mexican spot to eat. It was an important time for us. We needed that break after the doctors' appointment and before we went home. It was almost as if time would stop, everything would stop. We could just focus on being in the moment and being with each other. We didn't need to listen to test results or worry about when the next appointment was scheduled. It was no surprise after the transplant that food was on my mind again. First the popcorn, and then it was canned spaghetti and turkey hotdogs.

After three weeks in the hospital, I was sent home. I felt an immediate change in my health, though the pain of the swelling and the surgical incision pain were still prominent. I did eat meat for a short time after the transplant. It was a craving that I could not ignore, but I only allowed myself to eat turkey for a short time. I had a hard time satisfying my enormous appetite. My mom had an even harder time trying to keep up with it! I would be so hungry that she would be making food just about every hour. Mike, her date that she cancelled on the night we got the call for the heart, had stopped by the house to visit. They had kept on dating despite their first date being the night we got the call for the heart. Mike and Mom had their first two dates in the hospital when Mike came to visit and support Mom, any way he could. Mike brought a big box of Long Grove Chocolates and a box of doughnuts from the bakery where his eldest son, David, worked. I was sitting in the living room waiting for Mom to bring to bring me more canned spaghetti with sliced turkey hotdogs mixed in. She was in the middle of making it when the doorbell rang. I think I literally saw her go in two different directions at once that day. Amy and I were officially going to meet Mike for the first time and Mom, as well as Mike, was nervous about how it was going to go. "Meeting you two girls was terrifying for me!" Mike revealed that to us months later.

That damn Prednisone caused so many food comas; I couldn't keep up with my hunger anymore. It wasn't until much later on, that I would find out just how much of an affect the Prednisone actually had on my body.

CHAPTER 13

There She Goes

"There she goes, There she goes again
Pulsing through my veins and I just can't contain
this feeling that remains"
—The LA's

D
r. Mavroudis, a superbly talented surgeon, did a great job fixing my scar during the transplant surgery. He removed a lot of scar tissue that was left from when I had my fourth surgery with the pacemaker. It wasn't a long, red, raised, ugly, roly-poly like scar down my chest, but instead a nice symmetrical one that healed and faded as time went on. My schedule for the next three months was weekly biopsies, blood work every other day, and adjusting medications until the precise levels were achieved. Because I had episodes of rejection so early after being transplanted, more biopsies were required to make sure my anti-rejection meds were able to keep the rejection under control. Within the first couple of months, my anti-

rejection medication had to be changed. It wasn't strong enough to keep the rejection episodes from occurring.

I started out on Cyclosporine (Neoral), not to be confused with Cyclosporine which helps you "increase your tear production." Shortly after the rejection episodes, that medication needed to be reevaluated. Cyclosporine is very effective in other transplant patients as part of their regimen, but it wasn't strong enough to support my heart. Neoral and Prograf are strictly taken twice a day, as close to twelve hours apart as you can get, give or take a minute or two. Neoral specifically had to be taken two hours before a meal so it could get absorbed fully. Eating too soon after taking it would decrease the absorption and the full effect of the drug was compromised. It was imperative that I took my medication on time not only for the full absorption, it was also important when I needed blood work done to check the medication levels. If I didn't take them on time, the levels could be off and the results could be too high or too low. By now, I knew how important that was; especially when I was trying to make sure I kept from rejecting. A couple weeks after getting home and being on the Neoral, I started getting really sick. I was nauseous, throwing up and just feeling crappy. My doctor quickly switched me to another anti-rejection drug, Cellcept. Over the next few months my body slowly adjusted and the episodes of rejection stopped.

Mom and Mike were now seeing each other regularly and now they were an "official" couple. Mom was planning a time when we could meet Mike's three sons, David, Steve and Mark. All I could think was, "Well great, I have to wear a stupid mask everywhere I go now, and I am puffy everywhere." I was required to wear a face mask every time I left the house. It was so I would be protected from getting sick from the germs of other people. I got plenty of stares wearing that stupid mask. It was hard to ignore the looks from people, especially when you are already a self-conscious teenager. The mask and the swelling from the prednisone made it all worse. I tried not to let the stares bother me that much. I just tried to remember that most people looking at me would make up some story about it; they had no idea, really, what was going on with me.

We had plans to meet Mike's sons in the next couple of weeks at the mall. Mike never lets Mom forget how she had to cancel their first date because we got the call for the heart. Mike told people that he had heard all kinds of excuses about canceling a date like, "I've got to wash my hair." But never excuses like, "We are going to the hospital for a heart transplant." He would laugh about it for weeks and tell Mom they could have just put the heart in the refrigerator and kept it until Monday. I think it was their shared sarcastic humor that really drew them to each other. Mike never left. He fit in from the beginning. He was lucky because the three of us together Mom, Amy and I were a tough crowd!

In the summer of 1999, a popular art exhibit had made its way to Chicago, Cows on Parade. It was a collection of 300 life-size canvases shaped like cows. Artists were given a blank-canvas cow that they could paint with free creative reign. We had heard of the exhibit a few months before the transplant and had watched as the cows were put on display all over Chicago. Mom, Amy and I had been planning on driving around the city to see as many of the cow art statues as we could, but had yet had time to actually do that. I never felt well enough to go out, and I fell asleep every time I was in a car. The further into heart failure I went, the more I was sleeping, and we put our plans to see the exhibit on hold, like many things we planned on doing. We tried doing things and going about life as normally as possible when I was being worked up and listed for the heart transplant. It was already September and the last three months we still hadn't gotten around to see the exhibit, instead all we saw was the inside of the hospital. We had been in the city every week for doctor appointments, but never had energy left after those appointments to do anything, except maybe get something to eat. That wasn't any surprise.

Mom had mentioned to Mike that we all wanted to go see the Cows on Parade but never had time; nothing like the simple things in life that force a new perspective. It was two weeks or so after I was out of the hospital that we drove to the city to see the cows. I felt so much better after my new heart. I felt different. I felt healthy, truly healthy for the first time in my life.

The change in how I felt came so quickly. I still couldn't believe that this was how "healthy" felt. I was not lacking the energy like before. It had been exhausting to try and fight against my body and keep going physically. It was like gravity pulling me down with no choice but to give in.

I was still in pain from the surgery and from my migraine cycles. I was also dealing with the side effects of medication. And, I wanted to get out of the house so badly that I did my best to ignore everything until I got back home from the Cows on Parade tour.

I had finally gotten into the routine of taking my new medication and adjusting to being a transplant patient. It was a hard adjustment for me to make, but this heart felt more like mine than my own heart had. I still missed going to see Dr. Cole and Dr. Weigel for my checkups. I was down to about two cardiac caths a month and I was roughly two or three months post-transplant. School resumed and my tutors were back at the house at three-thirty every afternoon. Oh, it was so annoying to sit there and try to focus on history or math while fussing with my mask the whole time I was supposed to be paying attention. My friends had started their junior year in high school by the time I was able to start back with my tutors. I wanted to go back to school so badly. I was self-conscious about how I looked. Not because of my scar this time, but because I was so puffy everywhere and it was really hard for me to accept. Thank you "sweet" Prednisone, but I loathe you. I didn't even recognize myself, how was anyone else supposed to recognize me? I went from this little, probably less than 100-pound girl to a good thirty pounds heavier because of the medications. Naturally, I freaked out.

Mom took me to school for a short visit a few months later and it was so nice to see familiar faces and my friends welcoming me back. So many friends came up to me and asked how I was doing and how I felt. I often got the question, "Do you feel different having someone else's heart?" I could only answer, "I feel like myself." I felt different in the sense that I finally felt healthy and normal again. My new heart became a part of me instantly. The overwhelming feeling that I got from it was that this heart was meant for me. It was as strong and as much a fighter as I was, and we fit. Spending the time at school with my friends for those couple of hours made me want to get out of the house more often. We talked to my transplant doctors about me returning to school for my senior year of high school, and it was agreed that I could return.

Junior year was almost over, and I was looking forward to being in school even more for my senior year. There was no stopping my appetite, and I was thirstier than ever. I had never had a problem with extreme thirst before. I figured it was because I had been eating more foods that were salty; my thirst was trying to keep up. But, when you are drinking multiple bottles of pop, water or whatever you can get your hands on and the thirst does not subside, there is a problem. I was also moodier than usual. Admittedly, I am not always the calmest person, and I do tend to get into difficult moods for one reason or another. I had a schedule of appointments set for the next three months.

When seeing Dr. P and Carrie, they had gone through the same routine as we had since I got out of the hospital: EKG, listening to my heart and blood work to check my Cellcept and Prograf levels. Everything looked good. Carrie said she would call when my blood work was back from the lab, and we could make changes to my medication then, if necessary. The three weeks I had been out of the hospital had felt like months, I felt so good. The only exception was my thirst.

Another appointment finished, and Mom and I decided to stop at the mall on our way home. It was halfway between home and the hospital. We were shopping at one of the department stores and we hadn't been there more than ten minutes when I was hit with an intense feeling of thirst. If I wasn't drinking something excessively, I was running to the bathroom. I had never been someone who liked to drink a lot of water, and, not to get too graphic, my use of the washroom was normal.

We hadn't been gone from the hospital for even an hour when my mom's cell phone rang. It was Carrie telling her she needed to get me back down to the hospital as soon as possible. My blood sugar was dangerously high. She said she would explain when we got there. The only thing I could think was it didn't look like I was going to make it back home any time soon.

CHAPTER 14

Only the Young

"Look back in silence. The cradle of your whole life.
There in the distance Losing its greatest pride.
Nothing is easy, nothing is sacred, why?"
—Brandon Flowers

There was a good explanation as to why I was unable to keep up with the intense thirst and the feeling of needing to go to the bathroom every five seconds. Carrie told my mom that my blood test showed my blood glucose level well into the 700s. Normal sugar levels run roughly between 94 and 110, with small variations from person to person. I had never had any problems or mention of my blood sugar levels before. The look on my mom's face after Carrie had told her how high my levels were was nothing short of shock. I was admitted to the hospital within a couple hours. Numerous doctors and nurses were in and out of my room, continuously pricking my finger to track my blood sugar levels. I had been feeling a little cloudier lately.

Now, I wasn't sure what was going on, and I made it through these days not really knowing what had happened.

A cardiologist I had never met before came in to my room and told me that they needed to treat me for diabetes. I explained how healthy and careful I ate. He clarified to me that it wasn't necessarily what I was eating. Instead, I was told that it was a side effect of my new medications, though rare, that some patients develop after transplant. During the time I was being worked up for the heart transplant, the doctors told us about some of the possible side effects the medications could cause. They described the medication regimen would follow as part of my life and made sure that I would comply with it. They told us about the possibility of the meds causing nausea, diarrhea or excessive hunger and swelling from Prednisone.

Diabetes, though, was never mentioned. Because of that, we didn't know that the symptoms to watch for were excessive thirst and constant feelings of needing to urinate. We quickly found out those were symptoms of Type II diabetes. I was on a very high dose of Prednisone, and I developed glucose intolerance because of that.

At first, I kept running through events in my head, questioning myself about what I had done or could have done differently to prevent this new diagnosis. I had always been a healthy, careful eater and never had any problems with my sugar levels. In fact, post-transplant all I wanted to eat were carrots and celery. I did not understand where diabetes came from. Aside from that, I was very restricted with certain foods. I wasn't allowed to eat raw fruits or vegetables for roughly six months after transplant. Only fruits with thick peels like oranges and bananas were allowed. Grapes and tomatoes had to wait. Of course, that was all I wanted to eat. The saying, "You want what you can't have," really held true for me. Almost my entire diet was on the "do not eat" list, no celery, carrots or lettuce. In the last ten years, this rule about not eating certain foods might have changed, but I was told that those foods ran the risk of possibly carrying bacteria even after being washed. There was too high a risk that I could get sick from a virus or bacteria that was in or on the foods. I begged for at least three months straight for Dr. P to let me eat grapes, tomatoes and lettuce. When I was eventually allowed to eat those foods again, everything had to be washed multiple times before I could enjoy them.

"Can I see your finger?" I showed the nurse my finger, and, before I knew it, I felt a sharp jab as the nurse squeezed a drop of blood out onto a test strip. I was a sucker for that line. The nurse was tricky! She didn't tell me why she needed my finger, and I didn't question it. Hindsight is 20/20, and you can look back on any event or situation and say, "If only I had known." Clearly, it doesn't work that way. If it did, I would have known the signs and symptoms of diabetes, and then, maybe, I would not have been so surprised by this new development. It would have explained why I had felt so sick that Tuesday afternoon when Grandma and I went to lunch. Tuesdays, were our days to go to lunch and when Grandma didn't have a Mahjongg game to play. I had to eat what I felt I could keep down. The problem was, everything sounded good. At lunch, I had a gotten a small bowl of chicken noodle soup. I felt as if I was eating it in slow motion. My hands started to shake, and I felt like I was going to pass out, right into my small bowl of soup. Grandma immediately noticed the change in me eating to nearly throwing up over a period of ten seconds. She didn't tell me right away, but she said that she saw the color leave my face, only to be replaced by a pale greenish tone. I related it to just having a bad day and my body trying to adjust to my heart and medications.

I noticed my hands would get really shaky, exactly like the feeling you get when your blood sugar is low and you feel the need to eat something. The shakiness you feel all over your body is much like the feeling of being on the verge of passing out. This trembling got worse after I had foods or drinks high in sugar. If it had been low blood sugar (hypoglycemia), foods and drinks higher in sugar would have increased sugars in my body bringing me back to normal. If you are hyperglycemic (high glucose in the blood) the effects of eating or drinking sugary foods increases the symptoms because your body isn't getting rid of the excess amount of sugar (glucose, the same thing) from your system.

I was back in the hospital for another three days. It took that long for the doctors to get my sugar to a more manageable level. When they felt comfortable my sugar was under control, I could go home. One of the requirements before I could leave the hospital was to learn how to take my blood sugar and give myself insulin injections. The doctors prescribed Novolog 70/30 mix. In technical terms, it is a non-disease producing strain of bacteria that has been genetically altered to produce human insulin and has short and long-term acting insulin. I quickly learned how to test my blood sugar level with the blood-glucose meter. I was then able to determine how many clicks I had to turn the insulin pen, precisely injecting it and holding for ten seconds before removing, to make sure every bit of the medication was received. If you removed the needle right after you pushed the top of the pen, some of the medicine would squirt out; it did happen, several times. A dietician came in to explain what foods were high in sugar and what foods I could eat as much of as I wanted. She held up a chart that basically had bananas, apples, and grapes, oranges and fruit juices on it and then told me, "These are all foods you have to limit." Seriously? I looked at her and said, "That is basically everything I eat" (At least they would be once I was able to add those foods back into my diet). I loved grapes. Honestly, at that time, I loved everything I couldn't eat. Now I wasn't sure what I should eat. Maybe I would just stick with water!

My mom was standing next to my hospital bed, listening to the list of items the dietician read off. Chicken and turkey and other healthier white meats, I was told were fine to eat, and, for that matter, the dietician said I could eat as much of it as I wanted. I replied "I don't eat any of that." The only other thing I could eat as much of as I wanted was lettuce. Who wants to eat lettuce all the time? I asked the doctor multiple times if I could just take a pill instead of injecting insulin. Because my sugar was so out of control, the only way to treat it was by injection. The doctor told me an oral diabetic pill was possible in the future, but that depended on how I responded to the insulin injections first.

I had a rough time with the diabetes. It was an even greater adjustment than the transplant. Now, I was also having migraine attacks and visiting the ER at least weekly. I was put on several different preventative medications in particular Depakote, Reglan, and Motrin as needed, but nothing helped except the pain medication I got when I was in the ER. There was one day that I was scheduled for another follow-up cardiac catheterization through the groin, followed by six hours lying flat on my back. It was extremely painful to get up and walk after that much time, especially when I was trying not to move my head to keep the migraine pain from shooting through it. Oftentimes, I would end up with a terrible migraine after the caths, and I would literally be in severe pain from head to toe. This particular day, I had come back from my cath with a migraine. I was lying in bed waiting for the hours to pass and for the doctors to make their rounds so I could go home. The team stopped by my room, asked how I was feeling and I complained about having a migraine again and about the pain I was in. Kat was one of the nurses on my new team of cardiologists, and she had come into my room just after Dr. P and her interns left. She asked how I had been feeling, and I started to tear up in pain as I begged her for relief. She said, "We don't give pain medication." I asked if she could just ask Dr. P to allow me to take something, but she completely refused to ask on my behalf.

Instead, Kat looked at me and asked, "Jessica what's really going on?" I looked at her in complete shock and bewilderment, not understanding why she was asking me, "What's really going on?" The only thing I could say in between the pain surges from my migraine was, "What are you talking about? My head hurts, and I just had a transplant. I don't know what else I can tell you." She refused to accept my answer and kept pressing her question of "What is really going on?" I truly had no idea what she was talking about. I felt like she wanted me to say something like, "My mom neglects her kids." I had gotten a bad feeling talking to Kat. In fact, there were no problems at home. I had a rocky relationship with my father, and it wasn't at its best during the transplant, but that was the only thing I could tell her. She just kept pressing the question, and I did not know what she wanted me to say. Now I was in tears with a migraine and unable to move because I still had five hours left of bed rest.

Mom had left the room to get some food just before Kat came into my room and started interrogating me. When she came back about fifteen minutes later, I was uncontrollably upset. She asked me what had happened, and I told her about how Kat was questioning me and not accepting any of the answers I was giving her. She continued to harass me with the question of "what was really going on?" My mom was pissed off, and the look on her face was priceless. I think I literally saw steam coming out of her ears. You never want to make my mom mad especially when it comes to protecting us. She rushed out of my room so she wouldn't miss Kat before she left. She found her standing at the nurses' station with a couple of doctors. Mom told Kat in a tone that Kat would not soon forget that she was no longer allowed to talk to me without my mom being in the room. The way Kat had acted was totally uncalled for. Clearly, Kat didn't respect my mom's rule because she approached me a couple of times after that when my mom was not around. Once again, my mom had to "talk" to her, and it wasn't too much later that we began to have issues not only Kat but also Dr. P and her nurse practitioners. They were not a patient-first team.

I was doing really well with my new heart, but my migraines were getting worse. It was about a year after my transplant that I was in for a brief check-up with Dr. P and I came in with a terrible migraine. I was hunched over the side of the examining table ready to throw up and trying to be still so I didn't aggravate the pain. I was taking migraine medications that were not having any effect, but the doctor would not take me off them. I had been to see all the headache doctors to whom I had been referred, and nothing was helping. Dr. P came into the room and asked how I was feeling. I explained that I had another headache. She said to me, "Oh I get really bad migraines too. I take Excedrin." I thought, "Okay, you have got to be kidding me." I asked if there was something I could take, and she just brushed me off, as she often did. She said everything looked good, and I left upset. Compassion, attention and listening to her patients were not, by any stretch of the imagination, what my new cardiologist practiced. The next two years with her and her team were miserable.

I was going to see the doctor almost weekly, not because of my heart, but because my appetite was decreasing and I was having severe stomachaches. I am not one to make up stories about not feeling good, and yet, the medical team I now had made me feel like I was crazy. I was the patient who had all the rare side effects and complications, and I thought that they would have figured that out by now. But, I was wrong.

I had always completely trusted Dr. Cole and Dr. Weigel, and I did what they said to do. I never doubted that they provided only the best care possible. They were open to my opinion and input. I would try and wiggle my way around things I didn't want to do and sometimes they gave in.

With the transplant team it was so different. I knew it wouldn't be the same as with Dr. Weigel and Dr. Cole's practice, but I did not realize it would be so different and so hard. This appointment was the tipping point. My mom saw it from the beginning and she did not like it.

There are times when you just are stuck. We had nowhere else to go at the moment, as far as changing doctors. I was once again sick all the time. The diabetes took its toll, the migraines and now severe stomach problems were a daily obstacle. I thought that I had gotten through the hardest part, the transplant itself, but we didn't realize that the transplant was the easy part. There was still a really long road ahead and we had no idea how bumpy it was really going to be.

CHAPTER 15

I Am Alive

"All we do is not a lie and in the end we'll all be alright
But for now, I swear I'll try I really should be happy cause I am alive tonight"
—Test Your Reflex

There is nothing better than watching a good soap opera, especially when you can't go anywhere. *Passions* was the soap I watched religiously. If I happened to miss it, I made sure the VCR was set to record precisely at two o'clock. *Passions* was set in the small town of Salem. It had a quirky storyline with witches, the constant battle between good and evil, and spells gone awry. A witch was one of the main characters, at whom my mom often laughed. It wasn't lacking the typical soap romances, the tragic endings, and the many adventures of sabotage and relationships. It was obviously intended for a teenage audience. My mom used to watch *All My Children*, a much more dramatic and longer running daytime drama compared to *Passions*. Since Amy didn't get home from school until after *Passions* ended, I taped every episode every day so we could watch it together. Mom would be forced to watch with us when I was in the hospital. For us, those little things like watching a TV show helped to keep us moving forward.

As trivial as this might sound, it helped. At that time, it would have been really easy to give up on everything, particularly now with the addition of the diabetes and stomachaches. Having something that made us happy and gave us something to look forward to, was a small thing we all grasped tightly. We requested the movie *Meet the Parents* every time I ended up in the emergency room at the children's hospital. Every time that movie is on TV now, it reminds us of those visits. Actually, it reminds me of how the three of us would laugh together, even though we were in the ER. We still found humor even though I was in pain.

Between the ER visits for my headaches, sometimes throwing up uncontrollably, and having a difficult time finding anything that would stop or even control the pain and nausea, we ended up having more questions than answers. The transplant doctors couldn't explain why I was still sick and they were not really interested in helping us find a doctor who could figure it out. These complications weren't what transplant patients normally experienced, with the exception of rare cases of diabetes. The severe stomach pains were the newest symptoms I was experiencing. It felt like sharp stabs that pulsated constantly. Again, we had no answers. After many visits to the cardiologist with me lying curled up on the table, doubled over with pain, my mom said, "That's enough. Find someone who can figure this out." I was eventually referred to a pediatric gastroenterologist, Dr. L. He was hopefully going to help us figure out why I was having such bad stomach aches and throwing up everything; a sip of soup was even too hard for me to swallow.

First, I would need an upper GI endoscopy. I was given some very relaxing medication that didn't put me to sleep, but would leave me unaware enough that I wouldn't feel any pain when the tube was placed down my throat. At the end of the tube was a small camera in order for Dr. L to see if there were abnormalities, inflammation, or unusual masses in my GI tract. Fortunately, there weren't any signs of cancer. He did diagnose me with eosinophilic gastroenteritis that can be an allergic reaction to an unknown cause. "Extensive infiltration of the eosinophils" is what caused vomiting, mass pain, bloating, swelling of the abdomen and several other unpleasant symptoms. When I researched this type of gastroenteritis, I found that it is a rare and chronic disease with a combination of symptoms when an attack occurs.

Before this diagnosis, I had been made to feel like I was going crazy. I was constantly telling the doctors something else was wrong, and their response made me feel like it was all in my head when it wasn't at all. It was real. They would drag their feet when my mom or I would tell them that I was not feeling well. Eventually, I felt I was doing something wrong for telling them or felt like they thought that I was lying about it. Finally, with the concrete evidence that there was something very wrong going on, I felt a sense of relief. All I had to do was trust myself and listen to what my body was telling me.

New symptoms continued to develop. They didn't seem to be related to the gastroenteritis. This new and more noticeable pain radiated from the right side of my abdomen and around to my lower back. What was unusual was when I actually brought myself to eat some food; it would aggravate the pain, depending on what I was eating. I was told those symptoms, could be part of the gastroenteritis, and we didn't look into them further.

At this point, it may seem like all I did was complain without having any good things to say about these doctors. I am trying to be true to my experience and show that not all experiences are good ones. I trusted these doctors wholeheartedly with my life. I was optimistic and hung on their every word. They aren't bad doctors, but they were not a good match for me. There were known side effects from the multiple medications I was prescribed. When some of these side effects became reality and I complained about how I was feeling and the complications I was having, I felt like they viewed me as a difficult, crazy and/or uncooperative patient.

The high dose of Prednisone I had been on for a long time now was part of what helped in treating the inflammation and irritation of the gastroenteritis. I still have episodes of intense cramping and swelling. Since it is a chronic diagnosis, it will never entirely go away. At least now, I know what it is and I can take care of it myself without the help of a doctor or emergency room. Tylenol and carbonated water seemed to calm it down, make the pain bearable and have the attack finally subside on its own.

My problem with eating and keeping anything in my system was bad. I wasn't getting the nutrition I needed, and the only thing left in my system to throw up was bile—green, bitter, and very acidic bile. My mom and I sat and listened to what Dr. L suggested. "The only thing we can do is a feeding tube. We will insert a small tube in your stomach. You will be able to feed yourself through the tube so that nutrients can go directly into your system. It is the best thing for you." That was the ONLY thing he could come up with? I looked him straight in the eye and said, "No!" My instincts took over and I had a bad feeling that if I was to go ahead with a feeding tube, I would have ended up getting sicker. It wouldn't fix the real problems which were my stomachaches. I refused the "only option." I looked over to my mom to make sure she knew I was clear about my decision. She understood and agreed with me. She told Dr. L that this was not an option nor was it a solution. Plus, in my mind, it was going to be more trouble than it was worth. Another potentially painful procedure, the tubes and syringes that would be needed on a daily basis and then putting food or whatever through the tube so I could "get my nutrition." Dr. L wasn't happy at all with my decision. His next suggestion, which should have been an option along with the feeding tube idea, was to put me on a liquid diet. He would prescribe special protein powder that I would need to drink three times a day. It would help get me the nutrition I needed while calming and hopefully stopping the gastroenteritis attacks. Why couldn't he have just started with that? With more hesitation, I chose to try the shakes.

You may be wondering what happened with my Starlight wish. We made it to New York in March 2000, nearly seven months later. I hadn't realized how sick I was with my original heart. If we had gone to New York before I had the transplant, the time we actually spent enjoying the trip would have been minimal. I wouldn't have been able to walk around seeing as much as we did. I lacked the energy to keep up with all that Marci had planned for us. The timing of events worked out perfectly. They say timing is everything! I was so excited to see what Marci had planned for us that I had my suitcases packed two weeks before we left. Amy, my mom and her friend Barbara (who was supposed to go with us on the first attempt) and I got into the limo that was waiting in the driveway.

We went non-stop for the next three days. Mom had gotten us tickets for; *Annie Get your Gun* with Bernadette Peters and *Chicago*. We stayed at the four-star luxury New York Palace Hotel in Midtown Manhattan. The four of us sat in silence with our jaws dropping when we pulled up. It was amazing and beyond the point of luxury. We could not believe we would be staying here for the next three days. We didn't just get a room either. We got the biggest and most beautiful suite we had ever seen. None of us knew what to expect, but this was beyond anything I had pictured or dreamed. We took our time looking around the hotel, which was beautiful! It still had its old-world feel. It was called "the gem of Madison Avenue" so you can only imagine in the late 1800s, just shy of the turn of the twentieth century, how the extremely wealthy lived. It was turned into the hotel in 1980 and thirteen years later it underwent a multi-million dollar restoration project.

We were given our key card to our room and this was not just any standard room. It was an apartment minus a full kitchen. It was massive. Amy and I shared the master bedroom. Mom and Barbara shared the second bedroom. The rooms shared a large living and dining area. We were welcomed to the hotel with a bottle of Champagne, for mom and Barbara, and chocolate covered strawberries, chocolate chip cookies, fruit and bottled water. There was so much we wanted to do in the next three days, so we left our suitcases and headed out to walk around and start checking off our list of places we wanted to visit and eat at. Amy and I wanted to go to Mars Restaurant. We had heard about it so we had to try it (it was only in business a short time after that). They actually made the restaurant look like you could be eating on the planet Mars. The décor was red with moon rocks, craters and spacemen dangling from the ceiling. It was a fun experience. The one place Amy and I wanted to go more than anything was Serendipity III. All we could talk about was their frozen hot chocolate drink and how we had to try it. It was one of the best things I had ever tasted and the second I go back to New York that will be one of the first places I go.

Marci had gotten us tickets to see the Rosie O'Donnell show and actually be part of the live studio audience. At the time, she was like the *Ellen* of daytime talk shows, and everyone wanted to be a part of the live audience. We saw the first of two shows she was doing that day. They did one live airing and taped the second show that was going to air on TV the next morning.

Her staff was more than accommodating and very friendly. They asked me how I was feeling and gave us each t-shirts. I received a denim jacket with the Rosie O'Donnell logo. Her stage and audience manager escorted us down to meet Rosie after the show was done taping so we could get a picture and a quick autograph. We wanted to tell her about Starlight Foundation, that I had just had a heart transplant, and the wish I had made was to come to New York and do as many popular things that New York had to offer. To our disappointment, she didn't spend much time with us. She posed for one picture with all of us and quickly signed a couple of autographs before she rushed off backstage to get ready to tape her next show. My mom, Barbara, Amy and I all appreciated her time and said, "Thank you. It was nice meeting you and your staff," and we were on our way see more of the city.

The next day we happened to turn on the TV and the show Rosie had taped just after the one we were at, aired. Ironically, her guest on that show was Minnie Driver. She was on promoting her new movie *Return to Me*, about a young woman who was in need of and received a heart transplant in Chicago, no less. The clip they showed from the film showed places familiar to me that I had visited so often after my doctors' appointments: Lincoln Park Zoo, Michigan Avenue, and Grant Park. Minnie Driver's character had been through everything I had gone through seven months earlier. It still makes us all laugh when we think back on it. My mom will sometimes say, "We missed the show with Minnie Driver and that would have been the perfect reflection of recent events. Too bad no one from the show connected the two, it would have been really interesting."

We had so much fun visiting Times Square, Rockefeller Center, NBC Studios and then taking a full island Circle Line Cruise whose sights included the Empire State building, Brooklyn Bridge, Ellis Island, Statue of Liberty, and the twin towers a year before 9/11. We also saw Wall Street, Yankee Stadium and Central Park. Of course, one of my favorite places was Serendipity III where they filled goblets with ice cream and sundae toppings. The frozen hot chocolate was by far the most amazing thing I had ever had. We shopped in Soho and ate chocolate truffles in Rockefeller Center. Our trip to New York was more than I ever could have wished for. Marci and Starlight went above and beyond to make this trip memorable for all of us. As a result, I fell in love with New York.

CHAPTER 16

Brave

"Maybe one of these days you can let the light in
Show me how big your brave is
Say what you wanna say and let the words fall out"
—Sara Bareilles

D octor shopping" is a curious phrase, especially when it's used in a derogatory way. Why wouldn't you try to find a doctor who was going to listen to you and help you find answers to why, after a heart transplant, things weren't getting better? Dr. P had accused us, well Mom, of doctor shopping. It basically means that you, the patient, have several doctors that you are requesting care from at the same time, without any of the doctors knowing about each other. Sometimes this behavior is associated with people addicted to painkillers. They go see a number of different doctors to try and get multiple prescriptions. Each doctor believes they are the only doctor that patient is seeing and is more than willing to prescribe pain killers or whatever the patient is requesting to treat the ailment.

I couldn't understand why Dr. P would think that this is what we were doing. For one, they were the one and only transplant team we were seeing. I didn't even know of any other transplant doctors at the time. Because no one was helping us any further with my stomach problems, we were clear about wanting a second opinion. It is every patient's right to get a second opinion in order to find a doctor with whom they feel comfortable and believe they can trust. It is not an easy task to find even one doctor who would take on such a complicated case, let alone a handful of them. I was not looking for prescription drugs from any of the doctors and my mom wasn't either! The pain in my side and back went right through me taking my breath away. My mom insisted there was something more going on than the gastroenteritis, so she pressed the doctors to figure it out.

Then Mom had one of those light bulb moments during a conversation with a close friend of the family. She was telling her about her granddaughter who also had multiple heart problems. The friend told her that her granddaughter had had her gallbladder removed at the age of seven because it was causing problems. She went on to explain that her gallbladder was shriveled and the family was told that there was a connection between congenital heart disease and gallbladder problems. It was a long shot to even suggest it to the cardiologist, but everything my mom had read and researched seemed to make my symptoms a little clearer and point to something possibly being wrong with my gallbladder.

I went in to Dr. P's office for an emergency appointment a few weeks later. I saw the transplant nurse practitioner, Meg, who had known me for a long time before she worked with the transplant team. She had been a nurse on the cardiology floor, and I always asked if I could be put on her rotations when she was working. She was my favorite, and I knew she took great care of me. She always made me smile when she came into my room, even when I wasn't having a good day. So, I was beyond excited when she became one of the nurse practitioners for the transplant team. We knew each other well, and I thought she would be the one person who could help and who understood me.

I was doubled over in pain telling her the newer symptoms of the piercing side and radiating back pain. I couldn't eat anything, especially greasy food and foods high in fat. My mom suggested that we have my gallbladder checked. She went on to repeat what her friend had said. Mom explained that she, herself, had had gallbladder problems, which seemed to suggest it could be related to the congenital heart disease or a genetic factor. Meg said, "There is no reason to. We know you have gastroenteritis and that probably is what is causing the other pain." My mom turned, looked at me, then turned back to Meg and told her she wanted it checked anyway.

We assumed that Meg and the rest of heart transplant team knew that the immunosuppressive medications Prograf and Cellcept could cause gallbladder problems. Information about it was available on the Internet. To make sure for myself that I wasn't crazy, as every one of my doctors had made me feel, I did my own research as I have done throughout this book. I decided to google, "Gallbladder problems after a heart transplant" and "gallstones and gallbladder disease symptoms." Sure enough, there was evidence that it was possible after transplant that the patient could develop gallstones, biliary pain or colic. The University of Maryland Medical Center webpage gave me the best description. The majority of symptoms listed were ones I had complained to the doctors about for months.

I clearly remember Meg telling my mom and me, as we waited to see Dr. P it was true that the immunosuppressed medication could have an effect on my gallbladder. It was reassuring to hear her tell us that, but I didn't understand why everyone was telling us that it wasn't my gallbladder. That was the first of at least a half a dozen tests; ultrasounds, MRI's, x-rays, CT scans, stomach emptying tests, blood and urine tests. Every single test was negative, but the symptoms were only getting worse. They remained that way for the next two years.

Dr. W was my regular cath lab doctor, the one I requested every time I needed one. I got to know him and his dry sense of humor well. We respected each other, and I trusted him, literally, with my life. Mom and I went in one afternoon to see if we could get the results for one of my tests for gallbladder issues from Meg. She explained that nothing showed up on this test, much less any of the other tests that I had done. I will never forget it. I was with mom standing just off to the right of her. Dr. W was behind the check-in desk when Meg was going through every detail of what the test showed—no sign of gallstones. Dr. W's look was,

"You have got to be kidding me! You guys are back, and you keep making a big deal out of nothing. It is all in her head. My heart sank at the look on his face. As he walked away, he muttered to Meg and my mom, "It is probably just her menstrual cycle. It will go away eventually."

Traumatic was an understatement. These were the doctors that I had tried so hard to get along with and trust in. It had been a difficult adjustment for me from going from Dr. Cole and Dr. Weigel where I experienced a very loving and supportive environment to a cold and rocky one. I was a good patient. Hell, I was a great patient. I did almost every single thing that the doctors told me to do. I hung on their suggestions and longed for their approval and interest. I wasn't the typical, easy patient that they might have been used to. I had multiple complications and side effects that I really couldn't help. Believe me, if I could have, I would have chosen a far less complicated path then what it actually turned out to be.

I just could not understand why they wouldn't help. So what if the test showed everything was normal. Something was clearly not normal. The doctors said that if the tests came back negative, then there was nothing more they could do. Eventually, they tuned me out when they asked how I was feeling or if something hurt because my answer would be, "Yes, I don't feel good at all. The pain that is wrapping around to my back is unbearable. I can't eat, and I'm throwing up bile." I threw up bile when there was nothing left in my system to throw up (Bile is the acid that aids digestion, secreted by the liver and stored in the gallbladder that helps with digesting fats found in fatty foods). A common symptom of gallbladder disease is the inability to tolerate greasy, fatty foods. French fries, pizza, cheese, and pretty much any fried foods were bound to lead to an immediate attack. It helps in breaking down all the fats, and when the gallbladder is not functioning properly, it is unable to process these fats and the bile begins to work against the body because it has nowhere to go. I was told to try antacids to help with the acidity from the bile, which was normal. Normal? I don't think so. Many nights I would come down to Mom's office and tell her the pain was awful and I couldn't take it anymore. She didn't know what to do at this point and her only suggestion was to call the doctor on-call to see if he or she had any suggestions, at least for the pain. We had every possible test done to rule out gallbladder disease and, with each, we hoped something would show up to prove I was really in pain and my mom wasn't crazy for insisting that there was a problem with my gallbladder.

I would stand in the doorway of Mom's office as I called the transplant doctor on call. The doctor would call back an hour later telling they looked over my chart, and all they could suggest was that we head down to the emergency room. Clearly that wasn't helpful, and I knew that I would just get sent right back home without any more answers or help than I had gotten before. The last thing I remember trying to eat was green bean casserole. I took less than a fork-full before I ran to the bathroom sick and throwing up because the green bean casserole had touched my lips and instantly made me sick. It was close to Thanksgiving and I had been living with this pain for nearly two years.

CHAPTER 17

Angel

"Spend all your time waiting for that second chance
It's easier to believe in this sweet madness
oh this glorious sadness that brings me to my knees"
—**Sarah McLachlan**

We hadn't made much progress trying to get the gallbladder problem under control. My mom, the family and I were convinced that it was the gallbladder, but the doctors were convinced otherwise. Dr. L made it clear that he had no further help to provide us. He diagnosed the eosinophilic gastroenteritis, and, with that, he pretty much turned his back on us. There was talk amongst the doctors that I was a "trouble" patient and that my mom was only there to cause more problems. My mom was on a serious mission of looking for a new gastroenterologist in the Chicago area and soon got the name of one. My mom had a friend whose co-worker's husband was a doctor. He recommended a gastroenterologist at a downtown Chicago hospital.

Both she and her husband had high praise for this doctor and said that he would be able to help us. My mom gave the new doctor's office a call and scheduled an appointment for as soon as possible.

I had never seen a non-pediatric doctor before. Though I was considered an adult at the children's hospital, being nineteen, I was always reassured that I could be a patient with the doctors I was currently seeing until I was ready to move on. I was a passionate advocate and a proud patient of the transplant cardiologist and still would have been if it hadn't been for the last two years I was with her practice, suffering and fighting for everything I needed. I remember clearly upon my visit to the ER for another migraine telling the ER doctor that they needed to call my transplant team. I repeatedly said, "Call my hospital and my doctors." It made me feel good when I said that and I was naïve to think that would change.

My mom knew I couldn't survive much longer the way I was living. I really wasn't living, I was miserable, sick, and in pain constantly. We finally were on our way downtown for the appointment. It was my first experience with a doctor that was not in pediatrics. I graduated to the adult hospital world, yet somehow, it felt more like I was thrown into it. Dr. P. J. Kahrilas was willing to see me and take me on as a patient, but he told us he was not promising anything. All he could do was to try and help the best he could. He said he had another patient he had treated with the same symptoms and all normal results on their many tests, just like me. He said he suggested that they remove the gallbladder and the patient's symptoms subsided. Hearing that, my mom and I both knew he would be the one to figure out what the problem was. Dr. Kahrilas had my records sent over from the pediatric hospital, but he decided that repeating the tests would be best. Dr. Kahrilas did an endoscopy, colonoscopy, echo of my gallbladder, a stomach emptying study. Instead of being injected with a radioactive material through an IV line, I had to eat a breakfast of radioactive eggs! I was sitting in the lab where the test was going to be performed when I got a plate full of the eggs. The thought of eating was making me nauseous. It took me at thirty minutes to eat the plate of eggs. Once I finished, we had to wait a short time so the eggs could digest. I was turned nearly upside down and side-to-side to see how my digestive tract and gallbladder were passing the radioactive eggs. We would have the results within a week.

All the tests came back relatively normal. Dr. Kahrilas tried putting me on some prescription antacids (heartburn medication) to see if that would help with any of the symptoms. They didn't help to any great degree, but I did what he suggested. He told my mom and me, in all honesty, that the only way to know if it was the gallbladder was to remove it. While leaving that visit, he reassured me that, even though the tests were normal, removal wasn't completely out of the question. He said he wanted to do some research to see if he could get any information about my anti-rejection medications and a relationship to gallbladder disease. He called my house on a Saturday afternoon explaining to me that he had talked to a fellow doctor and explained my case, including the medications I was taking. This doctor informed Dr. Kahrilas that two out of three people who are immunosuppressed have gallbladder problems and the only way to see if that was causing the problem was to remove the gallbladder. Cellcept has listed side effects that could cause problems with the gallbladder.

I had started seeing Dr. Kahrilas towards the end of October and by December I was referred to a surgeon to schedule a cholecystectomy (gallbladder removal) So I wasn't crazy! Because it wasn't obvious and no tests came back conclusive of anything, it became an unimportant detail to Dr. P, her staff and Dr. L. With the reassuring, kind, honest, and willing-to help attitude of Dr. Kahrilas, we decided it was time to move on. We were finding another transplant team that could better support my needs as I got older. It was going to be much more convenient having all of my doctors under one roof, making a one-stop trip to the hospital. Aimee, a friend and fellow transplant recipient I had met a few years before at the start of my transplant process, told us about Dr. Cotts. She had since left the children's hospital and same transplant team I had had a few years earlier.

There were several major changes all happening at one time; new doctors, moving to a whole new team of transplant cardiologists and hoping that my having my gallbladder removed would make a difference in how I was feeling. My appointment with the surgeon who was going to be removing my gallbladder explained to us that there was a 50/50 chance that I would feel better once it was removed and I was willing to take that chance. He also said that two out of three patients that were immunosuppressed needed their gallbladders removed due to problems with the functioning of the organ that sometimes didn't show up on any tests. There was one catch, he said he would not schedule surgery until after he came back from his vacation. It was about a week before Christmas when we saw him and of course I was hoping that he would remove my gallbladder the next day, but really, my mom and I were hoping that we could get it taken care of before the holidays. Unfortunately the surgeon did not want to schedule the surgery before he left. He knew my mom wasn't happy that we had to wait until he got back from his vacation and he had made a note or mentioned to another doctor as we left that day, that I was going to end up in the emergency room when he was out of town.

Well, sure enough, I did end up in the emergency room...twice. I could not stop throwing up and now the pain stopped me in my tracks. It felt like overnight, everything got worse, enough for me to end up in the ER again. I was admitted to the hospital and spent another holiday season looking out a hospital window. The doctors tried to control the nausea and pain the best they could and scheduled surgery. Just after the New Year I was headed to surgery for a laparoscopic gallbladder removal. Dr. Shapiro was the surgeon since the one I was supposed to see was still on vacation. Dr. Shapiro was very friendly and compassionate. I only had three minor incisions where the laparoscope was inserted, removing the gallbladder through one of the three incisions. Dr. Shapiro explained the chances that they might have to create a bigger and more invasive incision if they found any problems with the gallbladder and perform the old fashioned way of removing a gallbladder with a scar that stretched from the right part of your abdomen to the rib cage (a five- to seven-inch-long incision). Luckily, the laparoscope removed my gallbladder without complications. Dr. Shapiro was great. I remember him coming to see how I was doing the next day. He only smiled and said, "Glad I could help!" It was a forty-five minute procedure; well for me it was two years and forty-five minutes.

It was almost immediate. The pain dissipated overnight and I woke up hungry—really hungry. Food sounded good again, and the thought of eating didn't make me want to throw up. The nauseous feeling was gone. It was surreal how fast the symptoms left after my gallbladder was removed. A few weeks after the surgery, we got a copy of the pathology report. It stated that my gallbladder was not functioning properly. Though there were no signs of gallstones or lesions, its function had been compromised. An unexpected and surprising bonus of having my gallbladder removed was that my, seemingly endless, migraines almost completely went away.

It had taken me a long time to accept that I was not crazy and there truly was something wrong. I learned a valuable lesson through both the heart transplant and the two years fighting for my gallbladder to be taken out, that the doctors aren't always right. I knew there was something wrong and my mom knew it too. Our strong gut instincts were telling us to not stop fighting until someone listened. We could have stopped, but the end result would not have been as desirable as just holding on and fighting a little longer. I guess the best way, the only way to get through it, is to go through it. Thanks to Dr. Kahrilas for listening to me and taking the chance to go ahead with the surgery and to Dr. Shapiro for removing my gallbladder, I was feeling better every day.

My thoughts were clear again and I could finally focus on going back to school. Only now, I was preparing to go to college. I was hoping that after high school and the heart transplant, I would be able to start college soon after graduating in 2001. However, the complications from the gallbladder put me two years behind. I had missed so much that it was overwhelming to start school again. I needed to ease my way back into school and I felt unprepared for college. But, I was determined. It had never been an option for me not to graduate from college.

I started at the local community college. After my first day of classes, I called my mom, crying and in a panic. I told her that I had no idea what I was doing here. I had been so far out from a school setting it was overwhelming. Mom reassured me that it would take time for me to get used to going to school and studying again. It really didn't take me long and I quickly remembered why I liked school: so many friends, new people to meet, new things to do and looking towards the future. I put all my effort into my classes, studying and doing well.

Amy was just about to start college too. During her senior year of high school she was able to take some early college classes at my community college.

The first class we took together was a speech class. I had been in school now for about a year and was working my ass off. I was intent on getting good grades.

Soon, Amy graduated high school, class of 2004, and was also working on her associate's degree. We spent those first two years studying and planning on transferring to a four-year university. We both made the honor roll several semesters in a row. Amy had won a full scholarship that covered her tuition and books for those two years. Our last semester at the community college was here. We were on winter break, at home with the family for our annual holiday dinner. My mom hadn't been feeling well for several weeks. I had pressed her, asking her what was wrong and if she had felt any better. She replied, "A little. It's just my stomach, I am sure it will go away. The night of our family holiday dinner, mom received a phone call around seven o'clock. It was a Friday night. Her test results from recent blood work and mammogram had come back and her doctor did not want to wait to tell her the results. She had been feeling more tired and knew something wasn't right. She hung up the phone, visibly upset. I asked her what the doctor had said and she said we would talk about it after dinner, after everyone had left. I instantly got a terrible, sinking, sick feeling. It couldn't have been good news because she would have said everything was fine as soon as she got off the phone.

Her results had come back positive for breast cancer. It was devastating. I cried uncontrollably on the couch in our living room with Amy. My mom tried to comfort us and tell us that she was going to be fine, but I just had no idea how to wrap my head around the news. Complete shock didn't even begin to describe my emotions. Mom explained to us that she wouldn't know the severity of the cancer until she went in for her lumpectomy. I felt like my world was crumbling at my feet. That clearing from the first dark storm that held all my medical problems was back. If you think lighting doesn't strike the same place twice well you are almost right. It strikes at least three times in the same place!

My mom was diagnosed with infiltrating ductal carcinoma (IDC). It was cancer, one of the most common and treatable type of breast cancer, but it was still cancer. I could not stop hearing those words. They are scary, toxic and uncertain—it is amazing how words can have such a profound meaning and effect.

The doctors removed the small lump revealed by the mammogram as well as some of the surrounding lymph nodes to see how far the cancer had spread. Thankfully mom had a successful lumpectomy and only one lymph node tested was positive for cancer. It hadn't spread past that to the other surrounding nodes.

The breast cancer itself was in the early stages. Unfortunately, the only way to treat it and take preventative measures was for Mom to go through chemotherapy and radiation treatments. I have severe anxiety when it comes to my mom or sister even having the slightest ailment, maybe because I know how it feels to suffer through significant medical issues. I would never want them to have to do that. They had already done it enough with me. I know my level of anxiety and worrying about the people closest to me getting sick, is unrealistic. It is some form of post-traumatic stress that I will have to deal with for a very long time. I just didn't know how to be the caretaker. I only knew how to be the patient. I knew it was incredibly hard for my mom and Amy to see me sick. Now, the tables were turned and I had a first-hand look at what they had seen for the last eighteen years.

My mom tried to tell Amy and I over and over again that it was going to be okay and that she was going to be fine. When mom couldn't calm me down (and that was rare) Amy could. Mom was telling me that everything would be okay even though she was scared and upset, too. She was reassured by her doctors that they had caught her cancer very early and set up a treatment plan. We barely had time to recover from all my medical problems when we were thrown right back into a medical whirlwind with my mom.

Here Comes the Sun

*"Little darling, the smiles returning to the faces
Little darling, it seems like years since it's been here.
Here comes the sun"*
—The Beatles

A my and I tried to focus on school as best we could while mom was going through her treatments. We would often take our homework to her chemotherapy appointments so we could study and stay with her. We were nearly finished with our Associate's degrees and were starting to apply to a four-year Bachelor's degree program. Amy was looking at few different schools including University of Illinois and Bradley. I knew I wanted to do something in business and entrepreneurship. Amy and I always had little businesses that we started, lemonade stands in the summer and selling jewelry we made. I set up a manicure table and painted Amy's nails, only to turn around and make her pay me a tip. In return, I made her coupons to use on her next nail visit. Entrepreneurship ran in the family. My grandfather founded Edgewater Rehab, a successful physical therapy practice and my mom had her own small business helping clients learn to speak better English with an emphasis on accent reduction.

DePaul University in Chicago and Bradley University in Peoria had entrepreneurship programs in which I was interested. I had a GPA of 3.6 and was just nearing the end of most of the requirements that were necessary to transfer to another college. I was confident that I had pretty good chance of getting into DePaul's College of Commerce and Bradley's entrepreneurship and business program. I expressed my interest in both colleges. Amy hadn't decided where she wanted to transfer to, but we had always talked about how we wanted to own and run our own business. We were not sure what kind of business we wanted one day, but knew for a fact it was going to be something in the food industry, and it was going to be ours! Amy and I both applied to DePaul University and Bradley. I instantly had a very strong feeling that DePaul was where I wanted to go.

We had been waiting for our congratulatory packages from the universities to come in the mail. We were so excited to find out if we had gotten in, especially to DePaul, or if we would come home to a letter that read, "We regret to inform you that you have not been accepted." I called my mom every day after class to see if anything from DePaul had come for us in the mail. We had just finished classes, and before I had a chance to call Mom, she called us. Amy was driving so I talked to her. "There were two envelopes that came in the mail from DePaul today," Mom told me. The first thing I asked was, "Are they the big envelopes or little envelopes?" You know that if you get a large envelope from the school, you are in. It is your coveted, "We are happy to inform you that you are accepted," letter and all the mandatory information about the school. The small envelopes however, are the, "Sorry you didn't make it, and good luck with your future applications."

Mom read my mind. I was just about to ask her if they were large envelopes she said, "They are the big ones!" I made mom repeat herself: "Yes Jessica, you and Amy both got large envelopes from DePaul."

We were dancing in the car the whole drive home, we were so excited. Our hard work had paid off. The fact that I had been out of school since high school and had managed to do so well in college was a huge accomplishment for me. It felt great! We still had a few weeks left of our last semester before graduating from the community college. Amy and I still went with mom to her appointments when we didn't have class. Mom would be finishing up her chemo treatments before we finished school. I wanted to be at every one of them, but it was nearly impossible to do that between classes, midterms and finals.

In June of 2006, we graduated. It felt like a graduation on several different levels. Amy and I were graduating with associate's degrees. We were getting ready to go to four-year universities, and Mom was graduating from her chemo treatments to just radiation treatments. Finally, I had graduated to a stable state in my health. Everything seemed to be cooling and calming down to a place where we could all catch our breath and relax. All the medical problems seemed to be under control now.

Mom, in her cute wig and all, had taken Amy and me to one of the last DePaul orientations before school started in late summer 2006. Amy had just turned twenty in May and I turned twenty-three in June. I couldn't help but have that overwhelming feeling I had when I started at the community college. It was scary to start something new all over again and now it was even bigger. There were a lot of major changes that were all happening at once. I was trying to keep up with it all. I was excited and knew what I wanted to do at DePaul, study business management and entrepreneurship. Our orientation tour guide, Jared, told us about the groups and clubs you could join. The one and only one I heard, and by that I mean paying attention to, was the Entrepreneurship Club DePaul Chapter. A second after he said that, I instantly knew I had to be a part of that club. My goal was to be chapter president. I never had the chance to be involved in any groups or clubs in high school, and I wanted to change that in college.

Mom had gotten through the worst part of her cancer the diagnosis, chemo and radiation and was doing really well. I was doing exceptionally well. People who had not known me before had no idea I had had any medical problems. I kept it that way for a while. It was time for Amy and me to enjoy our time at DePaul. We both became involved with the entrepreneurship club and threw ourselves into college life. We had found an apartment about a month before fall semester was to start in the South Loop two blocks from school: DePaul's South Loop campus, the College of Commerce. The people we met quickly became friends. They with were amazing and inspiring. Mike E., Rania, Ian, Alla, A.J, Chris Z., Robert D., and Brandon S. were a few of the people with whom we had become very close. To this day, I love and respect these people so very much. I feel I was lucky to have even more people in my life that looked past my medical issues and saw who I really was. Initially I didn't share my medical history with many people, but eventually this group knew the basics or the quick version of what I had been through. My explanation was: "I had a heart transplant when I was sixteen. It was no big deal. I am really good now," and their response back was, "Oh my goodness, really?" I always just smiled and nodded yes, then went back to whatever we had been doing; studying or getting ready to go out and have some fun in the city.

My professors never knew about my medical condition unless I had to miss class, which was rarely ever, for a cardiac cath that took me out of school for a couple of days. I prided myself on not making it an excuse. I was determined to make my own mark with hard work and dedication, not with pity and excuses. I still had a lot of baggage from the past that I hadn't worked through and it was still too fresh for me to talk about without getting upset. I wanted to be a normal student and be treated like every other student attending college.

Dr. Cotts had been my cardiologist for about three years. After Aimee suggested we set up an appointment with him in 2003, I immediately knew he was different. I had this overwhelming feeling of knowing I was in the right place. He was attentive, open, honest, and straightforward. He allowed me to have my own opinion and a hands-on approach in my care. He always took my ideas into consideration and would sometimes compromise with me on treatments. I rarely expressed opposition to what he suggested because I respected him and trusted him with my care. It was a drastic difference from my previous cardiac care. I felt reassured that Dr. Cotts and his staff were there for every single question and concern I had. He reminded me a great deal of Dr.

Weigel and his approach of patient care, which in today's world is unequivocally important in doctor-patient care.

We had a really good relationship after the first five minutes of our meeting and I knew he would take good care of me. I was far enough out from my transplant that I only needed to have a biopsy just once a year. At that time, if the biopsy came back positive for rejection, I would be treated with a short-term dose of Prednisone with a repeat biopsy in another six months. Otherwise, it was only a yearly occurrence. When my biopsies happened to fall on days when I had class, then and only then would I inform my professors of my medical history. I didn't want my absences to count against my grades.

I can't help but laugh at all the crazy college times we had with our friends. I admit, I did my share of partying and moderate drinking, but I was mindful of my doctor's recommendations and my mom's cautious warnings of being careful and not drinking too much. I was feeling great and wanted to have fun. Isn't that what you are supposed to do in college? Amy and I had the elevated train (the 'L') at the corner of our apartment building, making it very easy to get to different places around the city, like Lincoln Park, Downtown, Wrigleyville and countless other points of interest. Amy and I started to experiment with starting our own business. We had access to the Coleman Entrepreneurship Center at school where they offered free mentoring to students. It was perfect because we were beginning to form our ideas and goals around our own business, and the center was there to help give us direction in hopes of making our goals a reality.

We were in the early stages of developing a chocolate company: The Chocolate Rx, which we had dreamed up in November 2004. One day, I was in the bathroom fixing my hair, trying to think of a name for this business. For some reason I had picked up one of my pill bottles and the name kind of came to me in a light-bulb moment. It was only natural to play up on the medical feature, seeing as it was an immense part of our lives. It fit us so well and it made us so happy when we were in the kitchen creating.

Amy and I began experimenting, making chocolate creations out of our apartment. Many nights we would be up late, sometimes past three o'clock in the morning, making chocolate covered pretzels and Oreos. Raman and April, who worked at the Coleman Center, spent a lot of time helping us with our business plan, marketing concepts and listening to our countless ideas about where we saw the business going. In the meantime, we continued to study, get good grades, go out with friends and enjoy school like normal students.

I spent many hours working in a little sitting area where two oversized, reddish-orange chairs sat, just past the elevators outside the Coleman Center. Eventually, Mike E. would tell me he would meet me in my "office" because that's where he knew I would be. I knew exactly what he was talking about and laughed about it every time. We would share the office and hang out during passing periods before we were off to class.

Amy and I met Brandon in our Calculus One class. We rarely had classes together, but did share one every other quarter or so. We had the same prerequisites to fulfill. We met Chris Z. in Calculus Two. There is something to be said for friends and calculus. It's a good time to bond with people. Rania, Alla, A.J., Ian, and Liana were all a part of the Entrepreneurship club we were involved in. And Robert D., my love, we met in a one of our last quarters at school in a marketing IT class.

As ridiculous as calculus was, we had a crazy and fun study group. First of all, no one could understand the teacher due to his heavy accent. This would not have been so much of a problem if we had at least understood the math part of it, but that was impossibly confusing. Add them together (no pun intended), and it was a really tough class. It was one of only two classes in which I got a C in my entire college career.

Brandon, Amy and I had been in a study group together along with a couple other classmates. Brandon and I were in a group together in class and Amy, in another. Brandon would often forget to write his name on our homework, and because of that he wouldn't receive the credit. So, I would write it for him, and one day he turned around and said, "I could marry you for doing that!" I responded, "Put a ring on it!" from Beyoncé's song "Put a Ring on It" that was popular then. We would leave the room laughing and complaining about the new chapters of calculus we had to do. We laughed and joked around often about class and other random things. He made me laugh, helped me with calculus and ate the bags of chocolate covered Oreos and pretzels that Amy and I made for him and the rest of our calculous study group. Occasionally, Brandon, Amy and I would walk next door after class and go to Mondays for a drink so we could vent about how confusing the calculus problems were and how we had no idea what the professor was saying. I suppose if we hadn't goofed off, joking and laughing the whole time during class, maybe my grade would have been better. I doubt it though.

Our second, and last year, at DePaul was progressing faster than ever. I was evolving and discovering myself outside of the hospital scene, something that I hadn't had a chance to do in previous years. From a medical standing, my heart was doing great and my overall health was good. Switching to Dr. Cotts had been the best decision I had made and didn't have any problems under his care. He still considered my feelings about certain topics that would arise. He told all his patients that they should get the flu shot. Because of our already weakened immune systems, getting the flu without the shot might be worse than having had the shot. I listened to him and got the shot, once. I am convinced that created a flare up of rejection not long after. The biopsy I got that year was showing low-grade rejection. It was not treated, just carefully monitored. From that point on, I told Dr. Cotts that I wasn't going to be getting the flu shot anymore and he agreed with my decision. My point is that any good doctor will take all things into consideration and give you the best advice he or she possibly can. If you choose to go against it, they can only be supportive because it is ultimately your decision. These are some of the little things that mattered to me and that helped me trust in him. My mom was also happy with the care I had been receiving from all the doctors I had seen now that I was at a more mature, adult focused, hospital.

CHAPTER 19

Another Day

"There's only us There's only this
Forget regret or life is yours to miss
There's only yes, only tonight
We must let go to know what's right"
—**Jonathan Larson**, *Rent* the Musical

I realize that it is important to have doctors who have positive attitudes towards their patients. It helps their patients stay positive about their health, care, treatment and diagnoses and future outcomes. The only major medical issue that crept its way in, while I was still in college, was a pretty severe sore throat and sinus infection. For a little over a month, I was in seeing Dr. Chandra, an otolaryngologist (fancy name for a throat doctor or a doctor who deals with the anatomy, function and diseases of the ear, nose, and throat).

No one could figure out what was the cause of the soreness and irritation. I hoped that this doctor could figure it out. A couple of rounds of antibiotics and low doses of Prednisone didn't quite take care of the problem. I only had two quarters of school left, and I was hoping that this sore throat wouldn't last much longer. There was so much going on I didn't want to add another medical problem to the mix.

One night, our friend Jackie picked Amy and me up for a party. We all needed to take a break from studying for finals and figured a party was a good idea. On our way, Jackie asked both of us what our plans were for spring break. I didn't have any plans. I was just going to hang out and enjoy not having papers to write or tests to study for during the ten days of break. I was still struggling with the pain in my throat and found swallowing difficult and painful. Because of that, I had not been eating much. In addition, I was pretty concerned about my upcoming appointment.

I asked Jackie, our classmate and Amy's friend since grade school, what her plans were for spring break. She responded, "I am going to Germany!" I figured she was going for fun. Then she sprang up in her seat and said, "You guys should come too!" The idea was exciting. Amy and I had never been out of the country before. She explained that she was going to Germany for school. It was a class, not necessarily recreation. Studying abroad hadn't even crossed my mind. Amy and I both knew we wanted to be a part of this trip and we were somehow going to figure out how to go to Germany. We had just managed to meet the deadline to sign up for the class. It was a 10-week course, like all courses at DePaul, but over the ten days of our spring break, the class would be studying in Germany for an international marketing class.

We signed up for Prof. K's business marketing class the next Monday. We told mom that we were going to Germany later that day and began planning for our first trip out of the country. In a few short weeks, we would be off to Germany. This trip couldn't be all about the beer, Schnitzel and soft pretzels. Because it was a business class, we would be visiting some major German companies: Airbus, BMW and Ayinger Brewery. We were going to be learning about the production lines, the customers, the competitors and other operational and general day-to-day business operations. We would also have stops at the Dachau concentration camp and a Hamburger Sport-Verein football (soccer) game.

It was the best spur of the moment decision that we ever made. Every class trip like this is thrown together and the students encouraged to bond in a short period of time. You are spending nearly every minute together for ten days. It didn't take long before our group came together. We were an awesome group of twenty. We were leaving for Germany on March 17, 2008 only to return March 28, ten fabulous days later.

About a week before leaving for Germany, I had my first appointment with Dr. Chandra. I could not have asked for a better ENT. He was meticulous and cautious, and he took extra care in how he treated me because of my medical history. He explained that patients who have a compromised immune system are more susceptible to infections. I knew this but I didn't realize how sensitive I was to getting a sinus infection, nor did I realize how bad it was.

When I researched the side effects of the medications I was on and would be on for the rest of my life, I found that Cellcept (one of my immunosuppressive medications) could cause acute infection of the nose, throat or sinus. Dr. Chandra had a pretty good idea that my medications were at least part of the cause of the infection and probably the reason it had gotten so bad.

He ordered a CT scan that was done in his office. I had let the constant sinus pressure headaches go on for longer than I should have. I thought that with all the antibiotics and intermediate doses of Prednisone, the infection would have cleared up on its own. Having the CT in office was really nice because Dr. Chandra could give me the results in about ten minutes, instead of scheduling a separate appointment I would have to come back for on a different day.

Dr. Chandra came into the examining room with a bit of hesitation. He asked if I had been on any antibiotics and I told him that I had been on at least two rounds within the last couple of months. I could see the concern on his face. I think we were wondering the same question. Why hadn't either round of antibiotics taken care of the sinus infection? The CT scan showed that there was a severe infection that had taken over all of my sinus cavities. It needed to be taken care of immediately. I needed surgery and Dr. Chandra wanted me to have it done as soon as possible. As soon as possible meant that I was going to be scheduling surgery the following week, the same week I was leaving for Germany.

Before he could go any further I told him it would have to wait and I told him I was leaving to go out of the country next week. I had just gotten my itinerary for Germany and was packed and ready to go. Dr. Chandra's face went blank. I don't think he was prepared for me to say I was leaving the country. He asked if the trip could be postponed and he recommended I didn't leave. The infection was very serious.

I understood how serious it was, but I had no choice. Germany was paid for. He understood that and accepted that I wanted to wait until I got back from my trip to have sinus surgery. He was really worried about me going with such a bad infection and told me to check in with him before I left and as soon as I got back home. He prescribed another dose of a much stronger antibiotic along with some pain medication to help with the headaches. The surgery was scheduled for April 2. I did my best to ignore the pain and focus on enjoying the trip with our crazy, fun group.

We landed in Munich after a nine-hour flight. Our itinerary was jam-packed. We had so much to do and see, and we didn't stop. Germany has the same seasons as Chicago, so we didn't escape the winter weather. Luckily the wind chill in Germany is much less than back home. Munich was the first half of trip, and it was beautiful. The small, European, brick-lined streets, weaved through the city. Some seemed too small for normal-sized cars to fit down them, and they were. Motorcycles and Smart Cars lined the pathways, and rarely did we see a large sedan or SUV take up space on the streets. Prof. K wanted us to be "like the locals," which meant learning the S-Bahn and U-Bahn, the electric rapid-rail transit system, or subway. Our first assignment was to catch the S-Bahn, the Munich transit system, which took us directly to Marienplatz. Also known as St. Mary's Square, Marienplatz is the central square in the city Centre, home of the Munich glockenspiel. The glockenspiel is a musical instrument made of a variety of bells that are set to play a song. This glockenspiel, chiming clock, was added to the New Town Hall (Neues Rathaus) in 1907 and the chime could be heard every fifteen minutes throughout the day.

Marienplatz quickly became one of our favorite spots. It was easy to get to and it took us no time to learn how to use the S-Bahn and U-Bahn. We had some free time to explore the city in between our scheduled business visits. The sites, the history, the food and, of course, the beer were unforgettable. We spent half our time in Munich and the other half in Hamburg.

I did my best to not to think about how crummy I was feeling. I had days where it was still hard to swallow, and many nights where I couldn't sleep or breathe because my sinuses were so badly blocked. I was really good at keeping how I felt to myself. Amy was the only one who could tell when I was in pain and not feeling well. I hoped that when I got back home and had the sinus surgery, I could get back to breathing better with more restful nights of sleep.

Our last days were spent in Hamburg, the second largest city in Germany and the biggest port. We took a water taxi tour of the city and visited the beautiful Rathaus, Hamburg's town hall where the government is located. Rathaus offered amazing architecture that was built near the end of the nineteenth century. Farmers' markets, bakeries, chocolatiers, cafés and shops surround the town hall. Our business destination was Airbus headquarters. This plant plays a major role in the development and engineering of all Airbus aircraft and is where the final assembly of certain aircrafts takes place.

The infamous Reeperbahn, Hamburg's red light district was an experience. During the day, it wasn't so scary, but at night it was a different story. A group of us, along with Prof. K, decided to see what it was like when the sun went down. All we could do was walk as fast as we could, as close to each other as we could and not to make eye contact with some of the people who worked at the clubs. People tried pulling us into different clubs, which turned out to be strip clubs, and we all turned right around, exited and kept walking. It was one of the more unique experiences we had.

Our last day was spent at a Hamburg SV football game and it was a lot of fun. Before the game, we bought the home team's colors—blue, black and white—to wear to the game. It was unlike any sports event I had ever been to. The fans were hard-core. Anytime fans from the other team would cheer or boo, a fight would break out. It seemed to be typical and normal there. I am a huge Chicago sports fan and, a competitive one at that, but I couldn't keep up with the intensity of the German sports fans; especially when it was football, the most popular sport there. We had one last group dinner and then we packed to leave early the next morning. It had been an unforgettable trip, but I think we were all ready to get back home so we could catch up on some much needed sleep.

April 2, 2008 was upon me. It was a date that would become very significant and life changing in the year to come. I had no idea how bad an infection I had until Dr. Chandra told me he had not only cleaned out my sinuses of the infection, but also made some new passageways to improve my breathing and relieve the pressure. I was completely out of it for a while afterwards because of the anesthesia, so he had to tell me what he had found a couple of times.

The infection had nearly made it to my brain. If I had waited any longer to have the surgery, there was a good chance that the infection would have reached my brain and there was no telling how bad that would have been or if it could have been treated at that point.

Recovery from sinus surgery was one of the toughest recoveries for me. At times, I felt like I was suffocating. I would have panic attacks because I couldn't breathe normally. I had gauze and tape under my nose to stop the post-surgery bleeding. That was not at all fun. I had gotten sick several times due to the lingering effects of the anesthesia. I felt the pressure of throwing up in my head and in my cheeks.

Thankfully, I managed to miss only a few days of class. I was looking forward to my last quarter of college. It wasn't long before Amy and I, along with many of our friends, were attending graduation. The last ten weeks had gone faster than ever.

We took pictures backstage as we waited to line up and walk to our seats, waiting to hear our names called to go up and receive our diplomas. We tried to hold on to the last of our college life, promising to keep in contact with all of our friends while looking to what lay ahead for us in the real world. Fortunately we had Facebook to stay connected with friends.

In July, our lease was up on the tiny apartment we had shared for the past two years. We left remembering many good times and great memories. When we first moved into that apartment, I questioned our decision because of the fact that it faced the Metropolitan Correctional Center. But we were lucky to have such a nice apartment. It was a loft space and very conducive to sisterly fights. It was not exactly a great place to go and slam the door for alone time. Every word could be heard because it was a loft and the walls did not go to the ceiling. Friends spending the night on our air mattress and the smell of burnt popcorn lasting for days were just a couple of the memories we took with us as we locked the door for the last time.

Moving out and back home was a rough transition for Amy and me. And guess who got to drive the U-Haul? Me! Getting behind the wheel of that thing, one of the bigger trucks, and then having to drive it had its challenges. It's a good thing I didn't have to back it up! We packed up two years' worth of boxes and our little red couch that we bought when we moved in and headed back home.

In school we had focused our energy on trying to grow The Chocolate Rx. We figured out what worked and we focused on what we ultimately wanted to do in life. It wasn't exactly an easy thing to figure out. Amy and I seemed to have natural talents in the kitchen and it was the one place we were the happiest. I saw how Amy took over the kitchen and was fully enthralled in her work while she was there. We continued making chocolate for a while after we moved back home and managed to fill a few orders. It was an expensive endeavor and getting real paying jobs was the only way we could put more money into the business. Not only was it damned hard to find a job in the 2008 job market, it was also a hard task to find something that related to our major and was something we wanted to do. Our plan was to enjoy our last summer off, celebrate graduation, have fun and settle into living back home. We would find jobs in a couple of months.

Summer in Chicago is one of the best times to be in the city. The sun, the beach, concerts and street fests just added to the time we were spending with friends nearly every day. Cubs games were high on the priority list. Yes, we are all huge Chicago Cubs fans and have been since I was a baby! Nearly every Friday and Saturday night we enjoyed close friends, movies and food. We ended up seeing at least eleven new movies by the time summer was over. It didn't matter to us what we did. I was just so happy that I was able to go and do things and that I didn't have to worry about anything that related to my health and a hospital for a change.

Summer was passing by so quickly and I was grasping onto every last bit of time. It was nearly August and the pressure to find a job was mounting. I had been to the doctor only a few times for quick check-ups and the routine blood tests were status quo. A few times there was mention of a slightly increased Creatinine level, an indicator of kidney function. I was always told it was normal for a transplant patient to have a slightly elevated Creatinine level, there was nothing to worry about and they would keep their eye on it.

By late August 2008, I was beginning to feel a bit more tired than usual. I casually brushed it off with, "Maybe I'm doing too much and I'm not sleeping enough." The fact that I felt good outweighed any feeling or thoughts that anything could be wrong. All my doctors' appointments had been good and I was going to be going for my yearly heart cath with a biopsy in the next few weeks.

The job search was stressful and I attributed how I was feeling to that and to the transition from school to moving back home. It was a daunting thought and even bigger task to find something which I could be happy working at. Unfortunately, my expensive education was not helping me find a business-related job, and that was terribly disappointing. The job market was just starting to get really bad and I felt like I had failed at getting that good job I was supposed to get, the one I was expected to get, right out of college.

I began having stomach problems off and on that just continued to get worse. I couldn't say it was my gallbladder anymore because that had been removed a while back. It could have been acute flare-ups of the eosinophilic gastroenteritis, but even that was inconsistent with how I was feeling. Eventually the pain would subside. This pain didn't get any better and I was tired of going to doctors who couldn't tell me exactly what the problem was. I wasn't going to go back to the ER just to be sent home with a dose of painkillers, negative test results and doctors who were left scratching their heads as to the cause of the pain. I didn't have the energy for any of it.

CHAPTER 20

Pompeii

"But if you close your eyes,
does it almost feel like nothing changed at all?
And if you close your eyes,
does it almost feel like you've been here before?"
—Bastille

I was at that point again, the point where my mom said, "We need to go to the ER now and have this checked out." Amy, mom and I jumped in the car once again to head to the hospital. Of course, it was the weekend. It never failed that when I was really sick, it was always on the weekends or after office hours.

Nothing that I had taken helped control the stomach pain. I felt like I was drifting in and out of consciousness and that at any moment I could pass out. It was hard to breathe. With every breath I fought to keep my eyes open. To keep me alert, my mom kept asking me questions as we drove. My hearing was dulled and her voice came through so muffled I could barely hear what she was saying. I was panicking and trying to keep it from showing so I didn't scare or panic my mom and sister. It was a real challenge. I was really scared and I was telling myself to hold on, don't close my eyes and keep answering the questions even if nothing came out. Just stay awake. That half-hour drive to the hospital seemed like it was three hours long. I felt my body struggling to hang on, my heart was well beyond the point of racing and my mind was asking, "How the hell am I going to get up out of the car and walk into the ER", the thought wore me out. I tried to take deep breaths but even that was difficult. If I breathed any deeper I felt I would pass out for sure.

I don't know one emergency room that is actually efficient. People wait for hours to see a doctor for the emergency that brought them in and I am surprised more people don't die waiting. My pain was immense, it felt like someone was squeezing and stabbing my stomach, and the more I moved to try and lessen the pain, the worse it got. My blood pressure was high and my pulse racing. The ER nurse who was checking me in and taking my vital signs exclaimed, "Oh, your blood pressure is high!" No kidding! I am in horrible pain, ready to throw up all over you and pass out. Is that a good reason for it being high? She was asking me questions that I could barely answer. I mumbled that I was a transplant patient, but that was about it before my mom had to follow up with answers to the medical history questions she was asking.

There have been only two times in my life when I said to myself, "This is the end, but I don't want to die this way." This was one of those times. The other was when I woke up in the middle of the night, short of breath with very high blood pressure, just before I was diagnosed with diabetes.

At the end of me checking in, the nurse put a little color-coded sticker on my chart. As crappy as I felt or as out-of-it I was, I always would notice and ask the most random things. I asked why the nurse was putting an orange or red sticker on my chart and what it meant. At this point, I had memorized the colors of the little circular stickers that the ER used to code patients' charts. Each color represented a different level of severity of the patient's condition upon arrival in the ER. Unless you are transported by ambulance and you go right back to a room, you must rely on these color codes to tell you where you might be in line compared to other waiting patients. I believe that day the nurse put a red dot on my papers. Yes! Red was really good. The red (urgent) meant you were going to get in before the majority of the other patients. It would only be an hour to hour-and-a-half wait. An hour is nothing. In the meantime, I might have passed out while I waited. The next color is orange. It still represents an urgent patient, but one who can wait longer, maybe two hours. It's a toss-up. Blue and green are the killers. You have to wait forever. I am not sure how many days before you get in to see a doctor when you have that little green sticker on your papers. I can only imagine, though I assume you only get these colors if you have a broken bone or something similar to that.

The fight or flight response took over. I was fighting to stay alert, only allowing myself to relax a little after I had seen and talked to a doctor. I watched as people got called back to a room and was hoping I would be next. I am definitely not a *patient* patient! I had gotten up to see where my chart was in line compared to the other priority patients, but now I was hunched over in one of the small blue chairs in the waiting room and in too much pain to get up myself. I asked my mom to go up and ask how much longer it would be until my name was called.

A little secret of mine, though it really doesn't do much good on the wait time, is calling the doctor and asking them to let the ER know we are on our way. It is a good thing to do, especially if you are a transplant patient. They try and make your case a slightly higher priority.

Luckily my mom and I waited only about an hour before a nurse was calling my name to come back to a room. Mom had to help me change into a hospital gown. As I tried to lay down on the bed, the pain was so bad I could hardly lay still. It was in my stomach and the pain had expanded around to my entire lower back. I watched as the nurse put my IV in and pushed some much needed pain medication in to at least help. She drew blood and the doctor ordered a CT scan of my abdomen. She also ordered three barium glasses that needed to be consumed within half an hour. I was fighting now to not only stay awake because of the pain meds, but also not to throw up the thick barium drink I needed to drink to have a successful scan. I was more relaxed and able to sleep in solid fifteen- to twenty-minute periods, only to be shocked out of sleep when the doctor or nurse would come into the room. I didn't want to miss any new updates that the nurse or doctor might have had to tell me.

I kept shifting in the bed to try and find a comfortable position where the pain wouldn't be so intense. The ER doctor came right in and asked me the typical questions, "Why are you here in the ER today?" I wanted to say, "I am here for the fun of it and I enjoy wasting my time in the waiting room and being seen by doctors who don't believe my symptoms are real anyway." Okay, so I didn't say that, but I was thinking it. I told the doctor how much pain I was in, where it hurt and how long it had been going on. I don't remember his name but he was very nice and patient. He immediately said that he would get me something for the pain. I shook my head and softly said, "Thank you." He went on to tell me he wanted a CT scan of my abdomen and an X-ray because I was complaining of shortness of breath when I arrived. I waited for the nurse to come in with some pain medication. Thankfully, I was allowed pain medication every few hours. I looked at my mom and said, "They are going to make me drink that crap before the CT scan and I am not going to be able to drink it." I was brutally nauseated; not even water would stay down. My mom said, "Just relax. You don't know if that drink is part of the test." Sure enough the nurse came back to the room with a couple of bottles of the berry flavored Barium drink. My mom had already looked away as I shot her the, "I TOLD YOU SO!" look. I have been known to throw up after drinking that thick, chunky, chalky, white, berry-flavored drink that was necessary for the test. It coats the stomach and enhances any obstructions or places that might be bleeding in and around the abdomen. Before the test, I was supposed to drink two very full cups. I looked at the nurse and said flat out, "There is no way I can drink this. I won't be able to keep it down." She told me to do my best with it and to at least try and finish one cup. A worthy note: just because it says "berry" does not make the taste any better. Don't be fooled!

Five hours and a lot of pain medication later, I was disturbed from my nap when the doctor came in with the X-ray and CT scan results. The CT scan showed some inflammation in my abdomen that would likely go away in a few days. The x-ray showed something different. I had fluid around my heart. After they consulted my cardiologist, I would be admitted to the hospital so they could keep an eye on me. My blood iron and Creatinine levels were both abnormal and also a concern. The ER doctor then asked, "Have you ever been told your kidney function is abnormal?" I told him I had been told that they were watching the level. It had never really gotten beyond 1.3-1.5, so there was no great concern. It just needed to be monitored more closely than usual. My level was still within a relatively normal range, but teetering on the edge of where that damned red flag would be raised enough for the doctors to take notice. "Well your Creatinine level is around 2.3, and I have just talked to the heart transplant team and they want to watch you overnight."

I knew this was not good and one night was never just one night. I refused to be admitted. The ER doctor insisted that it was the best option and he had already talked to Dr. Cotts about it. I still refused and fought that answer with everything I could think of to talk my way out of being admitted. The only way I might change my mind was if I could talk to Dr. Cotts myself. If I heard him say I needed to stay then I would consider it. Sure enough, he called my ER room and sent one of his attending physicians down to talk with me to talk me into staying overnight.

I spent ten days in the hospital, but not for the stomach issues, which was the reason I went to the ER in the first place. It turned into watching my kidney function and relieving the fluid around my heart. The Creatinine level reflects how well the kidneys are functioning and 0.1-1.2 is a normal kidney function. My level was 2.3 and was continuing to decline. I was at about 50% kidney function. I also needed a blood transfusion to help with low iron. It took two pints of blood for the level to stabilize. This was my second visit to the ER for this issue. It was one of six visits there within a period of eight months and it was the first and only time in my life I had ever been sent home from a cardiac cath without having the actual test done.

After my heart transplant I had weekly and then monthly caths without incident. Never once was I sent home before the procedure was done. I was due for my yearly biopsy. It was supposed to be one of the last yearly biopsies before I could graduate to only having one every other year. I would be ten years post heart transplant that September and was happy with the direction in which my heart health was moving. I had great support from my doctors and I was happy with my care. It was exciting and motivating for me to get this one over with. I wouldn't need another cath for a whole year!

I was sitting in the waiting area where there were a couple of other recent heart transplant patients waiting for their caths, as well. There were more heart transplant patients than usual. I was often younger than the other patients waiting for their caths. One man asked, "What is a young girl like you doing in a place like this?" I explained that I had had a heart transplant and this was my yearly cath. He responded, "Hey, me too! My transplant was a few months ago." Another waiting patient piped up and said they were there because of a recent heart transplant, too. I had never really talked to any other patients waiting to go in for a cath, usually when I would overhear why they were there, it was not because of a transplant.

The day was really unusual. I didn't feel like chatting and was tired and annoyed that I had to be at the hospital at 6:30 in the morning. I was called back, I got my room and my nurse started my IV. An unexplainable feeling came over me as she was talking with me and preparing the vials for my blood work. I can't remember her name, but I remember her asking me why I was having this cath done. I had told her that I had a transplant almost ten years earlier. She looked at me and said, "That is just amazing. You are here for a reason and do not forget that." It was almost like I was talking to an angel. She made me feel calm and safe, which was rare for me at the time of my caths. I get very anxious and stressed when I go in for caths. It means large needles and pain for me, neither of which I like or do well with.

My nurse came in again to check on me and see if I needed anything while I waited for my labs to come back. The doctors can't start the cath without the results of the blood tests. The nurse turned to me again and said, "You are going to be okay." I smiled at her and she walked out of the room to see when the doctor would be in. Her words, "You are going to be okay," didn't seem to me to be about the test like what the nurses usually tell you. They say the test is easy, the doctors will take care of you and there is nothing to worry about. In fact, after what this nurse said, I felt like there was an invisible protective shield that surrounded me. It was weird. I sat back in my bed, alone, and just thought about her words. I could understand her amazement that at my age I'd had a transplant.

At the time I did not understand how valuable her words were and how I would hear them over and over again in my head in the months to come.

The doctor came into my room to explain the procedure, even though I already knew what to expect. He explained that they would be using contrast dye in order to be able to see the veins and arteries more clearly. He also explained the side effects of the dye and how the kidneys could take some time to filter it out after the procedure. Part of the procedure to protect them from the dye was to drink a coating agent. It smelled like rotten eggs and didn't taste much better.

The doctor finished his speech then excused himself explaining he would be right back with my labs results, as they had just become available. He came back in my room and said that he had some good news and some bad news. The good news was that I would not be having my cath done that morning. The bad news, the reason I wasn't going to have my cath done that morning was his concern with my elevated kidney function level. Simply, there was a decrease in the function of my kidneys. My Creatinine level was elevated and showed a decrease in function in the 2.3 range. My blood test showed the function level came back around 2.5 that, unbeknownst to me, was already getting close to my kidneys functioning at only 50%. The most important part of the test was the contrast iodine dye that was supposed to be injected during the cath so the doctors could highlight different tissues, vessels, tumors, inflammation or any other problems that would not have been visible otherwise.

Just when you think that you can't be shocked by what the doctors are standing there telling you, you can. The low kidney function level and getting sent home from a cath had left me speechless. If you know me, that doesn't happen often.

"What just happened?" I said to my mom as we walked out of the eighth floor cath lab, looking at each other, too dazed and confused to speak. Neither one of us could answer that question. When I did say something, I would stop halfway through my sentence, look down at my arm where the IV was pulled and just think, "OH CRAP!" We walked down the hall and around the corner to the elevators a short two hours after we first arrived. I knew this was not good at all. I had no follow up cath date. In fact I wasn't even allowed to reschedule it until Dr. Cotts saw me and we figured out what I needed to do next.

CHAPTER 21

If I Die Young

"Send me away with the words of a love song
The ballad of a dove
Go with peace and love
Gather up your tears,
Keep 'em in your pocket"
—The Band Perry

I was back in the ER a couple weeks after being sent home from the cath due to excessive throwing up with severe stomach and back pain. I knew instantly that I wasn't going to be going home that day and did everything I could to try and talk my way out of being admitted. I had been given more pain medication for my stomach and lower back and the doctors were doing the best they could to get me sent up to a room. I played musical hospital rooms. The doctors kept arguing on where to put me. The 13th floor was a normal floor, "normal" meaning not for transplant patients because there were carpeted hallways. The transplant floors have no carpeting anywhere because germs can be trapped there and even the slightest chance of germs could end up being harmful for a transplant patient.

It just so happened, that Dr. Chang, my internist at time, had heard that I had been admitted. He stopped in to see why I was in the hospital. I explained the whole situation and asked him if he was consulted about anything. To both our frustrations, he said he hadn't been informed that I was admitted and only knew because he saw my name on the board at the nurse's station. I told him I was being moved to the eleventh floor, the transplant floor, and that they were sending me to see a nephrologist. Dr. Chang had known something was wrong with my creatinine level early on when he called me after six o'clock one weekday. He was also the doctor who called to ask if any other doctors had seen how high my creatinine level had gotten and to tell me that it needed a closer look.

It would have been nice to know that this was one of the major side effects of the immunosuppressives I was on for my heart, the only things keeping my heart pumping.

This hospital stay was nearly two and a half weeks long. A couple of days in, the doctors informed me that I had a virus that was causing my stomach problems and that it would take time to make its way through my system. When I was able to keep food down, then we would talk again and see how I was doing and if I could then be released. There was barely any mention of my kidney function. I assumed that it was treatable with medications and the doctors would give me something while I was there to help my kidneys recover and gain a little more function.

Unfortunately, the next thing I knew, one of the doctors from the transplant nephrology team was in my room. I was sitting towards the edge of my bed, gathering strength to get up and walk to the bathroom to brush my teeth and fix my hair. My feet hadn't even hit the floor when Dr. Gallon walked into my room and asked how I was. He was tall with dark hair and an Italian accent. He was very nice and didn't waste any time asking me questions. He walked over to my bed, read my chart and asked, "Has anyone talked to you about needing a kidney transplant?" His cut-to-the chase questions caught me off guard and I looked at him confused. Well, confused doesn't even begin to describe the feeling. I responded, "No. Why?" He said, "Oh because you are going to need to be worked up for a kidney transplant." I tried to keep calm and just listen to what he said after that, although I have no memory of any of it until he said that it might be a year before I actually needed a kidney transplant. He explained that I would need to start seeing a nephrologist as soon as I was released from the hospital. They would watch my creatinine level, which had again increased to about 2.7 while I had been in the hospital. Dr. Gallon's team of three interns was waiting in the doorway for him to finish up his conversation with me. As they left, Dr. Gallon said from the doorway, "We will keep in touch and I'll see you soon."

The second that door closed I lost it. I burst into tears, panicked and tried to grab the phone with my shaking hands to call my mom as fast as I could. It was the one day she had taken off from driving down to the hospital. I had told her to, because no one needed to be there and watch me sleep the entire day. Besides that, I just wanted to be alone. My mom tried to understand what I was saying. "I don't know what's going on," I said between my tears. I am not sure how she could understand me when I didn't even understand what I was saying, what was going on, nor where the need for a kidney transplant even came from. I thought all I needed was to be monitored by a nephrologist for a while, nothing more. I tried my best to explain to her that I was officially considered to be in kidney failure. I yelled the word TRANSPLANT at her as if that was going to somehow make it less true. That word just screamed in my head over and over and I couldn't move. I told my mom I just had to go, I needed to go to the bathroom. She said she would call me back a little later and I hung up the phone.

I was hunched over the side, my head buried in my hands crying. I had nothing left in me to pull myself up out of the bed.

Before I got off the phone, Mom asked if I wanted her to come down to the hospital. She and Amy would come if I wanted, but I told her no, I didn't want them to come all the way down there just to sit and watch me cry. There was nothing I could do to change the situation. Having them be with me would just make everyone feel even more helpless, upset and confused. No one mentioned to me that another transplant was even a possibility. It wasn't until I was thrown well into the middle, that it became a reality. It was much like the way I found out about needing a heart transplant. And, for that matter, the only talk of a possible second transplant was during the heart transplant. There was a slight chance a second heart transplant would be needed if, for some reason, my new heart failed or was rejected in the very early stages of that initial transplant. That was understandable and part of the deal with organ transplants. There was always a small chance that the new heart might not be accepted or work the way it was supposed to. They did not inform us about the possibility of other organ transplants. We essentially had to start at the beginning and go through a transplant all over again. The only difference this time was I needed a new kidney.

I learned a great deal about kidney failure in a short period of time. Several things can cause kidney failure: diabetes (a leading cause), high blood pressure, trauma to the kidneys or some inherited and congenital disease such as polycystic kidney disease. I had diabetes after the heart transplant but that had been resolved for nearly seven years. I was told it was not because of my prior diabetes. My kidney failure was because of my Prograf. One of the two medications that were keeping my heart alive had attacked my kidneys. Prograf is highly toxic to the kidneys and over time can lead to complete renal failure (I use renal and kidney, interchangeably, as they both refer to the same thing). Even though I had received a visit from the kidney transplant doctors, I went to see my new nephrologist after I got out of the hospital. He told me that it could be a while before I needed a kidney transplant. I guess that was somewhat reassuring, the fact that it wasn't going to happen immediately. I had time to let it sink in a little and to come to terms with another transplant.

Amy had gotten a part-time sales job at the mall. I was looking for a job when Amy told me they still were hiring people. I took a job there as well, working as a sales associate, during October 2008. I had been feeling more and more run down, and it didn't help that I was on my feet for six to eight hours straight. As easy as that job was, you wouldn't think that it would be so tiring; for most people it wasn't. One night I was asked to fill in for someone in the perfume department. I walked over to one of the makeup counters and sat down on one of the stools where customers can get their makeup done. I wanted to fall asleep right then and there. That was the first time I noticed how much my lower back and feet hurt, with the exception of the last visit to the ER of course. I assumed it was from standing around for so many hours in bad shoes. The kidneys are located in the mid-back, just under the diaphragm and the lower ribs. When the kidneys no longer function the way they are supposed to, the excess fluid and waste material get trapped in the body, and have nowhere to go. The more fluid builds up, the harder the kidneys have to work, straining them and causing pain in the lower back.

Things seemed to just be getting worse. For those two months since my ER visit, I was in denial about what the transplant nephrologist had told me. Yet, the physical pain was evidence that what he said was true.

After the heart transplant, I stopped really talking about any of my medical history or what was happening. It was such a bad experience that I shut down and closed it off in my mind and completely refused to go into great detail about what happened during that time. I debated for a couple of days whether or not I should tell my friends about this next transplant. I would have to start back at the beginning and explain why I had had the first transplant. Most of my friends didn't really know about the heart transplant. I wasn't sure how they would react, much less how I would take their reactions, which was what I was more worried about. I didn't want them to pity me.

Only a few of my close friends knew I had been in the hospital, but I never really elaborated on why and what was going on. I was always hush-hush as I got older and just didn't want to face it, much less talk about it, after the heart transplant. Mom, Amy and I always had our own way of dealing. My mom told some friends and co-workers why she was missing so much work.

I finally decided that I would send a few of my closest friends a message on Facebook, explaining the recent events and what I was going to be dealing with.

Dear Friends:

I first want to say that I am so very lucky that you all are part of my life. I am so thankful for each one of you and love you all so much!!!

Most of you have a pretty good idea, if not know some of the health issues I have had in the past…Well for the past few months I found out that some of my heart medications were actually severely affecting my kidneys. I was put in the hospital in early September for an unrelated reason, but my kidneys were enough of a worry that they kept me for a week.

Come to find out, my kidney function is well below strong functioning levels. It is roughly at about 40% function (out of 100%). So...now the hard part...

I am looking at having a kidney transplant—hopefully not in the very near future, but more like in my time, which is about 4 to 6 months. I was told by my Nephrologist that I might have a couple of years before I would need a kidney transplant. But, the way things are looking right now I have a feeling that it might be sooner than they think.

This was a complete and total shock to me, as well as to my family. The thing that is the hardest is that with your kidney there is absolutely no indication of a problem until it is too late to do anything about it except have a transplant. Because I am a "special case" because of the heart stuff, things move even faster. What absolutely hurts me the most is I felt so great and amazing and healthy this summer, and just within the past two months things have changed. As of right now I have a clinic appointment on Nov. 21st. to start the process of seeing the kidney transplant doctors and being prepared for when the time comes.

I just felt like I needed to tell you all because I don't want any of you hearing things when it is too late. A few of you already know my feeling about the situation and have been truly amazing in helping me through some of this stuff. I thank you and love you so very much for that, and you are the greatest friends. YOU ALL ARE!!! I usually don't share this much information because I am used to doing what I have to do and then moving on.

At this point I am not happy at all at this situation and what is coming up, nor am I happy that I have a six hour clinic appointment...more like an info session on what to expect regarding your transplant...UGH. I hope that I will have at least a year before things need to be taken care of so I can figure out what needs to be done...I have a plan of what I want to do and so hate when things get in the way of that...

I think that you all know you mean the world to me and that, above everything else, all I want is to just be with my friends. I cannot say enough—you all are the best and I am lucky to have you all in my life for a lifetime!!!

Please, if you have any questions, do not hesitate to ask me or Amy...I kinda ran through quickly and outlined what was going on so I apologize if it is confusing. I know it is a bit shocking as well.

So much love to you all!

Within a couple of hours my friends wrote back with words of support and love. They left notes of encouragement and offered their help if needed. There was a whole ream of responses from them and it was overwhelming and comforting. I was so fortunate to have them in my life. I never doubted them. It was me I doubted, maybe because I was scared that I couldn't accept the reality I had tried to ignore for so long. Their reactions just gave me more strength. I had been so used to never saying anything about it. The people who I wanted to know did know once I hit that "send" button.

CHAPTER 22

You Get What You Give

"But when the night is falling and you cannot find the light, light
You feel your dreams are dying, hold tight
You've got the music in you, Don't let go.
This whole damn world can fall apart,
You'll be ok, follow your heart"
—New Radicals

Octuber was nearly over and my doctors had decided that I couldn't wait any longer to have my heart cath done. It had been months since that first attempt resulted in me being sent home without doing the test. Since my kidney function wasn't going to get any better, there was no point in waiting any longer. My schedule of medical procedures was as follows: a heart biopsy, another CT scan, and a kidney biopsy to see how much the kidney function had decreased. Once the heart biopsy was done, I could come back in for the remainder of the tests. Thankfully, I was not sent home from the heart cath this time. The cath lab doctors were well aware of what was going on and, though they used the dye during the procedure, they limited the amount to help lessen the work my kidneys would have to do to pump out the dye.

I recovered nicely from the heart cath. A few days later, the cardiac nurse practitioner called to ask me if I could make it down to my doctor's office the next day. They had made an emergency appointment for me to see Dr. Cotts at ten-thirty. I didn't really have a chance to say anything other than, "I will be there." What was I going to say? "No?" They didn't tell me much at all over the phone, so I wasn't sure exactly why I was rushing downtown the next morning. If it was rejection, the nurse would have let me know, and Dr. Cotts would have prescribed a round of steroids or adjusted my anti-rejection medications in order to get it under control. There was no mention of rejection or anything for that matter.

I told my mom I was going to see Dr. Cotts the next morning and she offered to take me. She would call work in the morning and tell them she was taking the day off. I just wanted to go and get back home as soon as I could. I didn't want her to miss a whole workday. My heart was great! There was no rejection and my immunosuppressive levels were right where they needed to be. I would only need an echo in the coming weeks. The main focus was my kidneys.

Dr. Cotts' nurse practitioner, Robert, rushed to catch me as I was walking towards the elevators to go home. "One last thing, Jessica…we have a room waiting for you upstairs. We have to admit you." I was standing in the middle of the waiting room, talking to Robert when he said this and all of a sudden I was staring blankly back at him.

"I was just about on my way out and you're telling me this now?" my very loud silent voice in my head that comes out in these situations yelled back. Dr. Cotts had made a last minute decision to admit me to try to bring my anemia back within a normal range. My labs from the cath had come back and showed that my red blood cell count was dangerously low and the only way to treat that was with a blood transfusion as an inpatient.

I was severely anemic. The most common type of anemia is iron deficiency. That was they type my doctors were trying to treat. But, there is also a type of anemia called anemia of chronic disease, an inflammatory disease resulting in chronic anemia such as a chronic condition like kidney failure. In either case, the production of red blood cells that don't yield the amount that the body needs to keep the bone marrow making the oxygen rich red blood cells.

I interrupted Robert, "I don't want a blood transfusion." I think I caught him off guard when I said that and insisted that I be admitted first and talk about what I was concerned about later. He said that they would also do a kidney biopsy to see where the function was . "Why do I need a blood transfusion, isn't there any other way to get my red blood cell count up?"

Unfortunately for me, there wasn't another option to get my red blood cell count up fast. A blood transfusion was the fastest and most effective way to do it.

I called my mom to tell her I was being admitted again and that my car was in the parking garage. I would let her know what room I was in. I also told her that I was refusing the blood transfusion. I was escorted up to my hospital room and the nurse started an IV. A doctor came in to talk with me and asked me to sign the consent form so they could start the two-pint blood transfusion. I refused to sign it and wanted to wait until my mom got to the hospital so I could talk to her about it. Within a couple of hours my mom got there and the doctors explained why the transfusion was imperative. I explained to her and the doctor that I did not want a blood transfusion because of a tainted blood scare incident when I was fourteen. The doctor said he understood my reasons for denying the treatment, but went on to explain, again, why it was immediately necessary.

It was about a year after my fourth heart surgery, when I was fourteen. The hospital called to inform my mom that blood from their shared blood bank had been incorrectly processed and cleaned. I had received blood during the surgery, so I was one of the patients potentially affected, and I needed to get a blood test as soon as possible.

It is the job of the blood bank technology specialist to type the blood and test it for disease. If the blood is free of disease, they label and store it until hospitals require it. Apparently the technologists responsible for properly testing the blood for diseases like hepatitis and HIV failed in that step. The blood that the hospitals and patients received had tested positive for HIV/AIDS. There had been one or two young patients who had already tested positive for HIV after they got blood transfusions during their hospital stays. The time period of the unused, recalled blood spanned a few years: 1996-1998. One of the labs that received the blood was at the hospital where I had had all my surgeries.

The only way to tell if I was one of the patients that was infected with the HIV virus was to have the blood test done. I was completely panicked about needing this blood test and there being a chance, even if it was one in a million that I could get the HIV/AIDS virus. We had learned a little about the disease in school and I knew it was a very bad disease without a cure.

My mom and sister were with me when they did the blood test. I asked the technician who drew my blood if I had HIV. I asked her what the symptoms were and how I would know if I had been infected. She explained to me that people who are infected with the disease show signs immediately and I would have already known if I had it. The reason she was drawing the blood was to make sure I did not have it. I was terrified and worried during the few days it took to get the results back and very luckily, my results came back negative for both HIV and the AIDS virus. Since that blood scare incident, there have been changes with new and stricter guidelines for the blood banks to follow.

I explained the whole story to the attending doctor. He assured me that the donated blood was put through a very rigorous process and that they had never had any problems before. The doctor explained to my mom that the benefits of having the transfusion far outweighed the risks, and they needed to get started as soon as I said, "yes." My mom assured me that it was going to be okay and that I just needed to let them go ahead.

It took a day and a half and a little over two pints of blood, to get my red blood cell count back within the normal range. After my levels were stable, I would be going down for the kidney biopsy. It was nothing compared to a heart biopsy. The kidney biopsy was relatively quick and I would be lying on my stomach. The doctor would insert what looked like a very long needle, into my back and snip a piece of my kidney tissue. It was a good thing I already had an IV in. I was definitely going to need some medication to knock me out for that test. I was insistent on that.

The doctor was kind enough to let me have medication and a moment or two for it to work before he started. I knew that needle was going to be quite painful. The doctor described every step to me as he performed it. First, he used an ultrasound to locate a good spot from which to take a sample of kidney tissue. As soon as he was finished with the ultrasound, he had the nurse give me something to relax me so that I wouldn't even know that he had done anything. Being on my stomach left me out of breath and my back pain continued to get worse and the doctor hadn't even used the needle yet. Before I knew it I was back in my hospital room recovering and preparing to go home the next afternoon.

The biopsy came back before I was discharged from the hospital and confirmed kidney failure. I was going to be seeing Dr. Batlle, my new nephrologist. When I met him, I liked him immediately. He would be keeping track of my kidney function and figuring out how they could keep my red blood cell count up without needing more blood transfusions. It was already November and I had seen Dr. Batlle at least three times. He suggested a new regimen that would keep my red blood cell count up as well as help protect my kidneys. The injection was Procrit and it was a ridiculously expensive medication. The cost without insurance was a few thousand dollars per injection. It is a man-made drug used to treat anemia, thus reducing the need for further blood transfusions by stimulating the bone marrow to make red blood cells. It was also intended to give me a little extra boost of energy, since that had decreased significantly over the last month. The insurance I had at the time wasn't happy about my being prescribed the Procrit.

At the time my insurance policy was with Humana. Right after I left my appointment, Dr. Batlle and his nurse submitted the claim to the insurance stating the reason I needed the drug. It wasn't 24-hours before Dr. Batlle's office called me back to say the claim was denied. Humana claimed that they had no proof that I was anemic enough to need such intense therapy and my doctors were to pursue other treatment options. Humana demanded my doctors prove to them they had exhausted all other less expensive options before they would consider covering the Procrit injections. Dr. Batlle and his nurse agreed to follow Humana's request but they did not give up on submitting claims over and over with proof of other treatments, in order to try and prove the Procrit was a medical necessity.

The one exception to getting the Procrit covered was to be admitted through the ER on a weekly basis. We were doing that and we didn't know how many weeks it would go on. It cost the insurance company more money than if they had just approved the injections in the first place. Hospitals charge for every Band-Aid no matter where you are or what you are doing in the hospital.

Before I agreed to do the Procrit weekly emergency room visits, I said I would try iron infusions to get my red blood cell count up. Humana was going to cover this because a doctor on their side had looked over my charts and suggested it. It would be a lot easier and would take far less time doing these infusions weekly as an outpatient. Every Tuesday I would check-in at the outpatient treatment center. An IV would be needed each time so the infusion could be pushed into my blood stream. Then about two hours later I could check out. The room was set up in an, "L" shape with large reclining, blue chairs lining the wall. Only six patients could be treated at one time. It reminded me of where my mom had her chemotherapy treatments: a communal room with nurses in and out, checking each patient's progress and asking them if they needed some water or a blanket.

By November I had to quit my part-time job. Between the numerous doctor visits and spending the rest of the time sleeping, I didn't have the ability to work. As simple as the job was, it was just too hard for me. I was at ten percent kidney function and officially in end-stage renal failure (ESRF).

Amy had been with me on most of these doctor's visits. She had heard the plan Dr. Batlle laid out and she thought the iron infusions were going to help at least for the time being. It also meant that Amy and I both knew that a kidney transplant was likely to happen much sooner than I was anticipating. I'm sure I remember Dr. G telling me that it could be a year or more so he wouldn't scare me any more than he had when he walked into my room and asked if anyone had mentioned a kidney transplant. Instead, we would be meeting with the kidney transplant team in the coming weeks. It was approximately two or three months since that hospital visit with Dr. Gallon. The need for a transplant in the next few years turned into needing to be listed and receive a transplant within the next few months.

I hated the iron infusions because they made me tired and sick. Obviously, they should have had the opposite effect, but the problem wasn't my anemia level. The iron infusions weren't going to have an effect on what the real problem was. After four infusions, I knew they were not making a difference. They were just making me incredibly sick. I would be in the bathroom throwing up a couple hours after the infusion.

There was, however, one and only one perk about the month I spent in the outpatient treatment center. There was a really cute guy who sat a couple of chairs down from me in the first chair in the row. The nurse who always took care of me when I was there noticed me staring at him as she was fixing my bag full of ugly brown iron filled liquid. She actually instigated the conversation. "He's cute, isn't he?" I said, "Yes, very cute." "Give me your phone number and I will give it to him." I laughed at the idea, but she came back with a small piece of paper and a pen. She went on to tell me, "He's single and lives in Chicago. He is going home to Ohio to visit his family and has two brothers." I smiled at her and told her I thought he was pretty cute. Amy was sitting with me at this treatment and she saw my wheels turning. Of course, I was curious, and I wasn't so out of it as to be unwilling to give him my name and phone number. It was a good distraction from my infusion that day and made the time go a little faster. Patient confidentiality kept me from asking the nurse what was wrong with him. But it didn't matter. He was a cute distraction, and I was more than okay with that. Amy, in her exact words said, "Jessica, you have the innate ability of focusing on guys that are either not right for you or are just a distraction." I can't exactly argue with that fact.

Humana denied the Procrit two more times, stating that my anemia was being caused by something else and continuing to fail to accept that my kidney failure was the cause. Dr. B and his nurses tirelessly wrote notes to the insurance to show that it was kidney related and that the other treatments were not making any difference in my red blood cell counts. They had been trying to get the medication approved for four months—October through January. Thankfully, Dr. Batlle had samples of Procrit he could give to patients when it was truly necessary. It was time for me to get an emergency injection before I left his office.

I had also refused to go back for any more iron infusions. They were doing more harm than good.

CHAPTER 23

Love Changes Everything

"Love, love changes everything
Hands and faces, earth and sky
Love, love changes everything
How you live and how you die"
—Andrew Lloyd Weber

T he fourth denial letter from Humana came in December. It wouldn't be until January that they finally approved the Procrit, deeming it medically necessary. Amy took me to see a lawyer about the insurance company refusing to approve the Procrit, but unfortunately there was nothing he really could do to fight it. He did send a letter to Humana stating that I had legal representation, and he was in support of what and how my doctors were treating my anemia. There had been some policy changes and major shifts in the takeover of Humana, which now had become Blue Cross and Blue Shield. January 1, 2009, Dr. B's nurse told me that Blue

Cross had approved the Procrit, and I could go ahead and finally fill my prescription for a six-month supply.

It was too little too late. I was going to start moving forward with the transplant process, again. Now, it was for a new kidney. I didn't have the one or two years before transplant that I thought I had when writing that Facebook message to my friends. In just three months, I was seeing the transplant team on a regular basis. My appointments with Dr. Batlle were slowly coming to an end. He and his team had done all they could for me in the last four months, which was mainly fighting with the insurance company for a medication that, if it had been made available to me sooner, could have changed a lot of things, or at least postponed things a bit.

Dr. Batlle and his nurse knew that it was only a matter of time before I was turned over to the transplant nephrologist. I didn't think it would be in just four months. Amy had been with me at almost every appointment. It used to be that my mom was always there, and now she wasn't there to hear every word the doctors told us. There was no sense in my mom taking off work to take me to these appointments when Amy could take me or I could manage getting there by myself. We would come back and tell her what was going on but to her it was never the same. Mom wanted to be there with us at these appointments, but there would be plenty of times when she would need to do that.

Amy and I went to meet the new transplant nephrologists. The same doctor that had told me I should prepare for a kidney transplant in the near future was at this appointment. I remember really liking him, despite the way we had first met in the hospital with him casually walking past my bed and saying that I was going to eventually need a kidney transplant. He was a genuinely nice doctor and explained to us what was going to be happening in the next few months. He was giving all this information, and I just nodded. Once again, I found myself not believing this was happening, and my reality felt strange. I caught one part of it as I was trying to stay focused on what the doctor was saying: "You will have to see if you have a living donor. The results are better compared to waiting on the list for a cadaver kidney, and the wait is a lot shorter." At that time, the wait list for a kidney was about five years. I didn't even think about a living donor.

Amy was my only blood sibling and asking her to be my kidney donor was out of the question. I did not want her to have to experience the pain of surgery or any of the tests that could cause her discomfort. I initially told the doctors that I did not want her be a donor. We had been at the hospital for a mandatory two-hour-or-so "information session", which would turn out to be one of several informative sessions that we needed to complete before I was cleared as a viable transplant patient, again. I told my mom and sister that I wasn't going to agree to the kidney transplant, and they looked at me like, "You have to do this, there is no other choice." In that moment, I agreed to it for my mom and sister. As for me, accepting to go through another transplant took a little longer. I needed to realize what the doctors were saying and face the transplant head on, despite my anger and upset.

There were still so many things I wanted to do in my lifetime—move back to the city, travel, get married, see Amy get married and have kids were at the top of my list. The thought of not going through with another transplant would have seemed like a selfish decision and an easy way out. That wasn't who I was, nor was I going to be that person. I never had been before and sure as hell wasn't going to start now. Do I wish things were easier? Sure, everyone does at some point. My life was my mom, my sister, my family and my friends. In those fleeting moments I sucked it up and just did what I had to do, back to reality. The only thing to do was to go forward. I was scheduled to meet with the social worker, nurses, nephrologists, and surgeons, much like I had done for the heart transplant.

Again, my mom had a hard time with not being able to be at every appointment with me as she had done for as long as I could remember. It was really hard for her not to hear every word the doctors spoke to us during all of the pre-transplant appointments. She knew the important stuff like the, who, what, where, when, why and how. I think that covered everything. Whatever I left out, Amy would fill in.

In one of the first appointments I had, Amy said she would donate one of her kidneys to me so I wouldn't have to wait five or more years to receive one. Her eligibility to donate would be determined through a series blood tests and cross-matching. Cross-matching was done after Amy's blood had been typed as

A, B, AB or O. Her blood was then matched to my blood to determine how compatible her blood and tissue were to mine. Blood compatibility has many aspects, and is determined not only by the blood types, but also by blood factors, (Rh, Kell, etc.). The more compatible the blood is, the higher the chance the donated kidney would have of being accepted by the recipient's (my) body, meaning that it would reduce the chance that the organ would be rejected. That is one of the main reasons why living donors, especially blood relatives, are successful donors. It also reduces the chance that the organ would be rejected and is one of the main reasons why living donors, especially blood relatives, are successful donors.

My initial meeting with the social worker seemed promising. It seemed like I would have a much better experience with her than I had had when I was going through the heart transplant. I told her how horrible that experience had been ten years earlier. I explained how no one listened to me when I was expressing my concern about how sick I still was and how upsetting and frustrating it had been for not only me, but for my family as well. I thought she understood right off.

I was seated at a small table in a small conference room. There was a line of patients waiting to talk to the social worker and the transplant nephrologist. It seemed like a job fair, the way they had the rooms set up and patients coming and going from room to room. The social worker I saw was well versed in my feelings of trust, or lack thereof, when it came to recounting the heart transplant process and that of Kat, who was only a nurse, and her actions of disrespect towards me and my mom. After all, you have to get through them before talking to the doctors.

I had specifically expressed to her how I felt that the last group of doctors who cared for me made me feel like my complaints about how I felt were ignored. They made me feel like it was all in my head and I wanted to try and prevent that from happening a second time. She assured me she would take care of me. I said, "Okay," and she gave me a hug, as if she had done something great and she was so proud of it. On top of everything, I was still having major stomach issues and now it was all related to kidney issues. The pain and lack of appetite were making things worse. I had gone to Dr. Cotts and he thought some of my stomach pain might be a reaction to the Cellcept. I had never had a problem with Cellcept before, but with all the changes that my body was going through with trying to fight renal failure, it was probable that I was having a reaction to it now. There wasn't much left to try in order to get the stomach problems under control. Dr. Cotts decided he would take me off the Cellcept and try another immunosuppressive called Imuran. The Imuran and Cellcept could be switched right away without any complications.

I had been on Cellcept for over nine years and was a bit hesitant to change half of the medication that was keeping my heart going. I was used to the Cellcept and knew that it was a good combination for me, but I decided to try the Imuran regimen to see if that made any difference in the stomach pain.

Unfortunately, the Imuran made things even worse. I was now eating even less and throwing up when there was no food in my stomach. I knew immediately it was the Imuran and insisted that Dr. Cotts switch me back to the Cellcept. I had only been on the Imuran for two or three weeks, but the change had been immediate and severe. I needed a final baseline cardiac cath done as soon as possible. The doctors were checking the coronary arteries to make sure there were no blockages (in heart transplant patients' coronary artery disease can occur much faster), right and left side heart biopsy (taking a sample of both sides of the heart to determine if and where rejection is) with the contrast dye. This cath was now just a part of the final kidney workup.

I had insurance. It was the same Blue Cross policy that had recently approved the Procrit. I wasn't initially informed about needing to apply for insurance through the state, which in Illinois is a Medicare and Medicaid policy. It was suggested, in passing, if I didn't have insurance I would need to apply for it, but I did have insurance. I had the Blue Cross/Blue Shield policy. We were going along with all of our scheduled appointments and doing everything we needed to do to get ready for surgery. Amy had her own set of appointments set up, being the donor and all. We did not have a date yet for the actual transplant. That came only after we knew for sure Amy was a match and healthy enough to donate, meaning she would be able to live with only one kidney. When her tests came back great, we were able to set a tentative surgery date for the end of February or early March.

CHAPTER 24

Better Days

"I wish everyone was loved tonight
And somehow stop this endless fight
Just a chance that maybe we'll find better days
'Cause everyone is forgiven now
'Cause tonight's the night the world begins again"
—Goo Goo Dolls

D id I say late February? February 25, 2009, to be exact, was the tipping point. It was the start of a series of some unfortunate events that would have me making some terribly hard, devastating choices. "Jane", the social worker, called me late that afternoon. I assumed she was calling because she had a couple of questions she needed answered prior to the upcoming office visit that was scheduled a few days later. That is not exactly where this conversation led.

She called to tell me, over the phone, "The surgery is off," and she suddenly stopped talking. My response was, "What!?" I was not at all prepared for those words. She went on to explain that "due to insufficient insurance coverage" I was not allowed to proceed with the surgery and the rest of the tests and blood tests that Amy and I needed to finish for the workup. Everything was to be stopped as of that moment.

Amy was sitting next to me on the couch when I took Jane's call. She instantly knew something was wrong when my voice became quiet and tears welled up in my eyes as I turned to look at her. There were insufficient funds. How could there be insufficient funds? I had insurance. Was the insurance denying the transplant, too? Of course the insurance was not denying the transplant; they covered the cost of it up to $30,000. They cover it all right, but once that $30,000 is gone, the remainder of the cost becomes the patient's out-of-pocket responsibility. Jane proceeded to explain that because there was a cap on how much the insurance company would pay for a kidney transplant, and because I was unable to pay the remainder (the cost of the OR, the doctors, the tests, etc.), they would not go through with the transplant.

Ironically, all of Amy's tests, surgery and hospital stays were free of charge because she was the one donating her kidney. The donors, thank goodness, are treated like royalty in that respect, as they should be, but the one who was dying would have to wait.

Jane, still on the phone with me, specified that the cost of the surgery alone would be upwards of $100,000. That did not include possible other treatments, blood tests, or clinic visits with the doctor. It was determined that I needed five plasmapharesis treatments to remove the antibodies, lessening the chance of rejection, just like I had before and after the heart transplant. Just one of those treatments costs over $30,000. Having one plasmapharesis treatment would wipe out the entire sum of renal transplant insurance coverage, and each treatment had to be billed to the insurance as a transplant-related expense.

I asked Jane what we were supposed to do. To my dismay, she did not offer up any help, comfort, advice or anything. Instead she said that until you are able to prove you have the money to pay the rest of the amount owed out-of-pocket, or until I enrolled in and got accepted for Medicare coverage, there was nothing she could do.

Medicare could take at least three months before I was approved, and I did not have three months. Where was this information when we first started talking to her and all the doctors about needing the kidney transplant? That should have been the first thing we did, but no one said anything to us about it. Jane also explained that, "You could live on dialysis for a long time if it were necessary." She acted like it was no big deal. Dialysis is a big deal. It is a definite life change and I wasn't ready to live the next five years or possibly more on dialysis. I couldn't understand how Jane could be so cold and unresponsive to my being upset, especially when her job was working with exactly these types of situations. She was a social worker. Aren't they there to help the patient? I guess she missed that part in school because she was neither a support nor a help. "Until you can prove you have the funds to pay for all costs involved in the transplant or you get Medicare/Medicaid, the remaining appointments and surgery date are postponed."

I was in tears when I hung up the phone and Amy was not far behind with her feelings. My mom had come in to the living room and saw we were upset when she heard all the commotion, me yelling at points during the conversation.

Everything we did from that point on was because we sought out the help and resources ourselves—well; my mom and Amy did. I had no idea what I was supposed to do. My mom told me that she was going to contact our state representative's office, Mark Kirk at the time, to see if there was anything he could do to help. Unbeknownst to me, Amy had gotten on Facebook not long after I got off the phone with Jane. She sent a quick message to some of our closest friends. In fact, I had no idea she had reached out to our friends for several days. This was the message she sent:

"Subject: NEED HELP ASAP!!!

Hi,

I'm sure most of you know that Jessica needs a kidney transplant and she will be taking one of mine. Unfortunately we have had some major problems with insurance and have hit another bump in the road. I need to figure out how to raise some money

ASAP. If any of you know how to do this through Facebook or know of someone who knows how to do this let me know. The insurance will only cover $30,000 and the whole transplant will cost over $100,000. The rest we will have to pay out of pocket, which we definitely do not have. The hospital will not move forward if they don't think we can pay for the transplant. She cannot wait another 3 months for a kidney.
    PLEASE let me know!
    Thanks so much,
    Amy"

We have some truly incredible and amazing friends! Within the hour, we had responses of advice. A.J. was the first one to reply, saying that he had gone to a launch party for a new fundraising organization called GiveForward. They were a new online company that helped users create fundraising pages for a variety of things for which people needed to raise money. There were several cancer fundraiser pages, people raising money for vacations, for marathons and a variety of other causes and activities. The point was to help people raise the money they needed so they could do something they otherwise wouldn't be able to. A.J. gave us GiveForward's contact information.

I had been out with a friend the whole day. When I got back home my mom stopped me in the hallway just as I was going into my room and asked, "Did you know what Amy did for you?" Know what? I had no idea what she was talking about. I was out of the house all day and hadn't talked to my sister except for a few text messages back and forth.

I had a hard time just sitting at home. I had a hard time being anywhere. I felt trapped in a body that was no longer working the way I needed it to. It got so bad I wanted to crawl out of my skin some days. The day after I talked to Jane on the phone, I just needed to get out of the house.

CHAPTER 25

Time After Time

"If you're lost you can look and you will find me,
Time after time If you fall I will catch you, I will be waiting
Time after time"
—Cyndi Lauper

B efore I left that day, Amy was sitting on her bedroom floor hunched over her computer. She occasionally worked on her computer while sitting on the floor. We had done that all through school. We would spread out our homework and have our computers on the floor instead of working at our desks, so I didn't think anything of it. I went into her room to tell her I was going out for a while and asked her how the new black coat she bought for me looked. She knew my style better than I did, sometimes. She and mom asked me if I was sure I was feeling good enough to go out. I assured them I would be fine. I'd be back soon and told them that I loved them.

Only my mom and Amy knew exactly what Amy would be doing on her computer for the next three hours. She would be setting up the fundraising page on GiveForward. When I got home and found out what Amy had done, I was in shock.

GiveForward is a personal online fundraising site founded by Ethan Austin and Desiree Vargas Wrigley. Ethan graduated from American University with a law degree but found a greater love of helping people to actively raise money any way he could. He would do it by running in marathons or wearing his famous banana suit, raising every penny he could. Desiree graduated from Yale University. With GiveForward she wanted to create a place where people could have more of a say in where their money went when it was donated. It would give them more donation options and change the way people viewed donating.

Amy had an active fundraising page up on GiveForward's website by that night. She spent over three hours filling in all the "required information" fields so she could publish our fundraiser page. She reached out to the "ask for help" section on the webpage and Ethan got back to her immediately. In the beginning, Ethan, Desiree and a few interns were the only people working at GiveForward who could help with fundraising questions and concerns. Ethan and Desiree were there every step of the way for us. Amy talked to Ethan almost every day since starting the fundraising page and he had been personally involved in helping Amy with our fundraiser. He was a lifesaver. Desiree was, too. There were no two better people for this job. Both Desiree and Ethan were the most compassionate, caring, focused and driven-to-do-good people.

Ethan told Amy that if there was anything we needed to just let him know, and he would do whatever he could to help out. Amy updated the fundraiser page daily. One of the best features of the site is that it allows the users (creators of the fundraiser) to update information as needed and as often as possible. It allows donors and potential donors to read updates about the fundraiser. That made it more personal and real.

When Amy started our page, we were the first medical fundraiser on the site. It was a learning experience for Ethan, Desiree and us. We had never done fundraising like this, and GiveForward had not yet had a medical fundraiser like ours that brought a lot of attention and funds to the site itself. There were other fundraisers where the donations went to cancer research or other causes like that, but ours was different. We were to be the first successful medical fundraiser on the site so far. Amy had set it up asking for help to pay for the remainder of the medical expenses that were expected to total $100,000 or more, the amount we needed to come up with before we could schedule another transplant date.

Amy named our fundraiser, "*Help Jessica Get a New Kidney.*" Ethan, Desiree and Amy posted the link to each of their Facebook pages in hopes it would gain more attention and donations. Hadn't she done enough by saying yes to being my kidney donor?

Once that, "publish your fundraiser" button was clicked, I couldn't take that information back, it was out and people could read about everything. I had been closed off from talking about anything that related to my medical condition. I didn't realize how much I was in denial about everything since the heart transplant. I don't remember ever feeling like I couldn't talk about that kind of stuff. My mom was always very good about being open with me when I was little and encouraged questions. Because the heart transplant was so sudden and was truly a rough time for me, I think I decided I was better off not talking about it. When I did have to talk about it, I was very basic in my explanations. I was adamant about not wanting to be viewed as "that girl," the girl who had the heart transplant. People judge and assume they know you based on words. Sure there was something greater than words here, but I just couldn't deal with it.

When I found out about the page Amy created and who Ethan and GiveForward were, I had no choice but to face my medical circumstances head on and ended up talking about everything. After all, if I couldn't accept them, acknowledge them and not define myself as, "that girl" no one else would be able to do that either. It started with me, although Amy became the catalyst for the much needed change in my attitude. Before I could say anything to Amy about the fundraiser she told me that they had already started to receive donations almost immediately after publishing, "*Help Jessica Get a New Kidney.*" It had not been 24 hours since starting the page before donations started showing up on the page, some with messages of love and encouragement attached. There were donations for twenty dollars, ten dollars and then one for $5,000 showed up that read "anonymous."

Amy was overcome with emotion and unexpected joy when she came back to her computer and saw the donations pouring in. Ethan and Desiree were just as surprised as we were by the response. The generous donations kept coming: friends, family, friends of friends, and people we didn't know donated varying amounts of money. No donation was too little. Every penny was greatly appreciated and would have an amazing impact on us.

March 4, 2009, I once again found myself in the ER. I had been having some trouble breathing with minor chest pains. I had let a couple of days go by before I decided to tell my mom how I was feeling. I wanted to wait to see if the pain would subside and my breathing would go back to normal. I thought it could have been stress especially with the aggravation the kidney transplant was posing. The only reason I did eventually tell my mom was I wanted to make sure nothing was seriously wrong with my heart. There was always the possibility that my body could shut down when there were other organs that were failing. That situation puts more pressure on your other organs, making them work harder than they normally would. Of course, the thought that my heart could be affected to the point that I could be rejecting due to the failing kidneys made going to the ER very necessary.

The ER doctor ordered a chest x-ray. He could hear with his stethoscope that there was some fluid in my chest, but he wouldn't know the extent of it until he had the x-rays in front of him. I knew that this visit to the ER was going to end up with me being admitted to the hospital.

While I was waiting for the test results, Amy and my mom went to talk to the hospital's patient representatives to explain how Jane had called us and told us over the phone that the kidney transplant had been cancelled until further notice. I was so tired and barely could respond to what Amy had come back and told me in my ER room. I remember nodding my head sluggishly. I was grasping for small breaths at times as I tried to rest, but there was just the feeling of pressure on my chest that made doing anything difficult.

I am not sure when mom and Amy got back to my ER room but they must have gotten there just before the doctor walked back in to tell me I had fluid around my heart that was causing the shortness of breath and pressure. My kidneys weren't able to push the excess fluid out of my body, causing fluid retention. The ER doctor started me on diuretics to try and get rid of the excess fluids. A woman from patient services called up to the kidney transplant department and spoke with Jane after mom and Amy had talked with them. Two hours later, still in my ER room, Jane had called down to talk to me. One of the nurses told me that I had a phone call they were going to put through to my room. Mom and Amy had been back from speaking with the patient reps for a while now, so it wasn't either one of them calling me.

I had been given medication to treat the fluid buildup, as well as some pain medication. The nurse came into my room to tell me that she was going to put a call for me through and that I needed to answer it. Jane needed to talk to me. I remember asking, "Who?" as the morphine haze took full effect. I could not figure out why Jane would be calling me in the ER, and, for that matter, I wasn't in the mood to talk to her, especially if I was going to hear more bad news.

I reluctantly picked up the phone just after the nurse transferred the call to my room. Jane proceeded to explain that it was decided that the transplant was back on. After I was admitted and settled into a room, someone from the transplant team would be around to talk to me about my new schedule of appointments.

Just two weeks earlier she was telling me they had to stop the transplant, and now it was all of a sudden back on track. I didn't believe Jane at first, and to make sure I had heard her correctly, I asked her to tell my mom exactly what she had just told me. It was just in case I had heard her wrong or had dreamt what she had said. She got on the phone with my mom and told her the same thing she had told me. Mom repeated it to Amy, who was sitting in the chair right next to her, with a smile on her face and a look of relief.

I wasn't sure what changed their minds to go ahead and get back on track with the surgery, but mom and Amy explained to me later that, though it would take some time for the paperwork to go through, I was automatically going to be approved for Medicare. By explaining this to the patient services rep, the rep then talked to the team and explained what was necessary to get things moving again. Just about a week before this hospital visit, we found out that if you are in end-stage renal failure (ESRF) you are immediately eligible for Medicare coverage. For three years Medicare would pick up the remainder of the cost of the transplant.

It would have been far less upsetting had we been given Medicare information, regarding ESRF, in the very beginning. The doctors say they don't deal with the insurance portion so they couldn't have helped. Jane should have known and explained how Medicare would be a necessity. Then there would have been no insurance issues in the first place, and the transplant wouldn't have been stopped. Unfortunately, it wasn't surprising that we had to find it out for ourselves far later than we should have. We had Mark Kirk's office working on getting the approval on the Medicare so we could show proof of insurance. In the meantime our fundraising efforts continued. The hospital knew about the fundraiser Amy had set up and knew that there was a little money to access if needed. That was also part of the reason the transplant was on again.

CHAPTER 26

The Heart of Life

You know, it's nothing new
Bad news never had good timing
Then, circle of your friends
Will defend the silver lining
—**John Mayer**

A ll the ER visits were getting redundant. Be admitted, go home, go see the doctor for a follow up, then be admitted by doctors' orders. I was in the hospital from March 3 to March 16, 2009. We were now hoping that we could set another date for the surgery while there. About five days into my stay, a doctor mentioned dialysis. The one and only time I met her, she was telling me they wanted to start dialysis as soon as possible. I thought I would be able to avoid dialysis, but instead I was told that I needed to seriously consider it. Before the doctor could finish her sentence, I said, "No!" and turned my head so she would leave me alone. Before exiting the room she told me, "You need to seriously consider starting dialysis as soon as possible. You can have a little time to think about it, but there is very little time." The fluid was building up around my organs with nowhere to go.

The fundraiser had been going really well. Amy and Ethan were talking almost every day, trying to figure out who in the media they were going to talk with next, about what was coming up in our fundraising efforts. Ethan had gotten in touch with several of his contacts at newspapers and in TV and radio.

We were still getting nowhere with the hospital as far as financial assistance, a payment plan or anything that would get us a scheduled date for surgery. Within the next month we had articles in the *Chicago Sun Times, The Chicago Tribune*, health blogs, DePaul Online and on WBBM radio. March was a busy month. Ethan connected with Amy with Steve Miller at WBBM Chicago. Amy's interview with Steve Miller was aired March 9, 2009. I was still in the hospital, but was able to listen from my hospital room.

Here is a transcript from the radio interview Steve Miller conducted with Amy

> *Woman Raises Surgery Money to Donate Kidney to Sister*
> *'Steve Miller Reporting*
>   *WBBM) - Thanks, perhaps, to the power of the Internet — and a sister's love — a 25-year-old Chicago area woman is getting a kidney transplant sooner rather than later.*
>   *No stranger to hospitals is 25-year-old Jessica Cowin.*
>   *She had a heart transplant ten years ago. And now she needs a kidney transplant.*
>   *Her 22-year-old sister Amy has volunteered to donate one of hers. But Amy says Northwestern Memorial Hospital would not perform the surgery because Jessica's insurance for transplants had been maxed out ten years ago.*
>   *"I figured if we raised at least $100,000, we could give that to them and they could go ahead with it sooner."*
>   *However, a spokeswoman for Northwestern says, "Jessica was neither denied nor told she would never be transplanted; she was informed that she needed to wait, (because) at the time, the status of her health didn't warrant*

immediate transplanting... Jessica and Amy are to be commended for their tenacity and proactive stance in attending to Jessica's health needs."

Through Facebook and www.giveforward.org, Amy started raising money.

"Within less than two weeks, we've raised $24,000."

Amy Cowin says Northwestern has agreed to perform the transplant surgery.

We'll never know exactly what the tipping point was."

The fundraising continues for medical expenses. Transplant surgery expected in the coming weeks.'

Time wasn't on my side. We couldn't sit around doing nothing, especially not Amy. Being in action also helped me focus on something other than how I felt and worrying about things I couldn't control. It was some kind of movement towards a resolution, one for which I was so desperate. Another day passed and I was still adamantly refusing dialysis. The same doctor who had come to "talk" to me about dialysis had followed up to see if I had changed my mind at all. I told her I was going to wait until my mom got the hospital later that day. The doctors didn't know how much longer I was going to need to stay in the hospital and they wanted to make sure they got me into the procedure room for the port. I finally said okay.

I needed a port put in in my upper right chest area so the nurses and doctors would have easy access to do dialysis. It would also be used for my plasmapharesis treatments. The port was semi-permanent. I would have it in until sometime after the kidney transplant. It also eliminated the need to be poked for an IV every time I went to plasmapharesis treatments or dialysis if and when I chose to do it. Actually, it was the only way the medicine could be administered during these treatments. The rate of the flow from the fluid that flows in and out of the tubes is high and had to be given through the arteries in the chest. The veins are too small for that much fluid to pass through. They would blow, or collapse, if it was done using IVs. It would cause more damage than necessary.

Mom had finally gotten to the hospital and the doctor wasn't far behind. The doctor explained the reason for the port and the necessity for me to have dialysis as soon as possible. I understood the reasons, yet I couldn't help but think this would never have been an option if the transplant hadn't been cancelled. My mom reasoned with me, "If you have fluid building up around your kidneys and can't get rid of the excess yourself, what are you going to do when it happens again?" It made sense as the doctor was saying it, but I was still very reluctant to say yes. The doctor further explained that the fluid buildup was becoming a problem all over my body and the only way to relieve the build-up was to remove it through dialysis. I ached all over and my skin was painful to the touch, which was eerily similar to when I was taking the large doses of Prednisone after the heart transplant. I hated having that feeling again.

Later that night I decided that I would allow them to put in the port the next afternoon and start dialysis, though with great hesitation and resentment. I was so upset that it had gotten to the point that I wouldn't make it to the transplant without needing dialysis. I couldn't stand hearing the word "dialysis." Everyone knows what it means. It means you are sick, really sick, and aside from a transplant there is nothing more you can do.

There were only a few things that cheered me up, and one was when friends came to visit. Two of my close friends stopped by the hospital to see how I was doing. Chris Z. came by on his way home from work one night and it was nice to see an outside face. I filled him in on what the doctors were telling me and what tests were coming up in the next few days. I asked him how his day was, what he had going on the rest of the week and his plans for the weekend. I was happy that he had come to visit and appreciated him coming and keeping me company. It gets pretty boring in the hospital after, well, about an hour. I had always been reluctant to have visitors, so it was a nice change for me to allow them to come.

Later that week another good friend, Robert D., came to see me in the hospital. He recently reminded me about that visit. He told me that he was not at all good with being in hospitals. He had had to sit down for a minute before he entered my room. He didn't like the smell and sounds of the hospital; they made him dizzy and sick. I kind of giggled at that because I had no idea about that when he came to visit. I didn't remember him saying anything about not feeling well. When he came to see me he brought a little stuffed toy dog. It was so sweet and comforting and the dog stayed with me the rest of the time I was in the hospital.

According to medicine.net the formal definition for dialysis is: "A medical procedure that uses a special machine to filter waste products from the blood and to restore normal constituents to it." My personal definition differs a bit: simple hell, but includes a patient confined to a machine for four hours unable to move about freely and seated alongside a row of other chairs waiting to be filled by more patients.

I was scheduled for the port procedure soon after I had relented. They fit me into the schedule the next day, and it was supposed to take less than an hour. The doctor explained the procedure. Typically the area where the port was to be placed was numbed so when they made a tiny cut in your chest with the surgical knife, it wouldn't hurt.

After I heard, "numb the area" that was it. I told the doctor, "You better just put me out for this. I don't want to feel anything. If that can't happen then I will not let you put in the vascath (port)." It wasn't like the doctors could run back to my mom for permission to override my decision. I was still capable of making decisions and this time it had to be done my way. One way or another, I wasn't willing to feel the pain of this vascath being put in; my skin cut, pulled and pushed to fit the catheter through the small incision near my collar bone and then the sewing of the four stiches that were needed to keep the line in place. The doctor continued to explain what he was going to be doing after the incision had been made. A small plastic tube would be fed through that tiny incision in my chest and then inserted in an artery and a vein. Both the artery and vein needed to be accessed during dialysis.

The doctor was very nice and told me he would make sure that I was put completely out for the whole procedure to ensure I didn't feel anything he was going to be doing. I looked at the nurse, nervously, and she confirmed what the doctor had just said. I felt a small sense of relief and a little less anxious.

I woke up back in my room, groggy from the medication with my right arm perched on a couple of pillows. My back was stiff and I tried to push myself up to change positions trying to relive some of the back pain. Within seconds I felt a rush of pain that ran down my shoulder all the way to my fingers. I didn't expect it to be that bad. I just about jumped through the ceiling in pain, began to cry and pressed the nurse call button. I tried to look down at my chest to see what the port looked like. All I could see was a big white bandage with two small plastic tubes, one red and one blue, sticking out. Then I noticed how badly I had bruised. I followed the black and blue marks all around the site of the port, up to my shoulder and about a quarter of the way down my arm. Tears were rapidly flowing down my face. It freaked me out to see the tubes sticking out of my chest and to feel pain so bad I could barely move my arm. I don't know if it was because of the pain or because of what I had just seen. My reaction was about the same as it was when I was thirteen and saw my scar down my chest for the first time. I was disgusted. The nurse came in a few minutes after I pushed the call button. I told her I needed something desperately for the pain. First, she helped me carefully adjust my position in bed so there would be less pressure on my arm and shoulder. A couple of pillows under my arm helped a bit. As she was fluffing the pillow she said that she would be right back with some pain medicine. When she returned, one of the residents on call followed. Now that the port was in place I could start dialysis immediately. I was going to the inpatient lab within the next couple of hours.

Amy followed me up to the dialysis lab. Patient beds were parked all around the room. There was room for about six hospital beds. Two or three beds sat to my right. I was in the corner spot and parked at an angle so I could see off to my left side as well. It was like a drive-in restaurant where you pulled up to order, park, wait for your food, eat and leave. My food wouldn't be ready for at least five hours. The first treatments always took longer because of the amount of fluid that was built up and how fast the doctor wanted the machine to run. I was up there around five hours. I had heard that it could be upwards of six hours or more, depending on how much waste and extra water needed to be removed. All that would be monitored throughout the stay, as well as how well I tolerated the machine. My arm and chest around the port were brutally sensitive. The nurses needed to be very careful when they were hooking me up to the dialysis machine.

The blue line removes the blood, which contains the waste, extra salt and other materials that cannot be removed on their own. The red line returns the cleansed blood back into your body. Heparin is used to prevent blood clots, given at the beginning and end of treatment.

Though this was not funny at the time, this story makes Amy and me laugh every time we tell it. Amy was planning to stay with me in the dialysis lab until I was finished or until my mom arrived at the hospital. I had told the nurses to keep an eye on her for me in case I fell asleep. Amy had been sitting in a chair against the wall, just across from my bed watching the nurses prep me. The next time I looked over, about five minutes later, she was gone. I was, of course, concerned and asked the nurse where my sister had gone. She said she would find out for me. Plus, Amy would have told me if she was going back to my room to hang out and wait for mom. Another nurse had overheard me ask where my sister was, and she volunteered, "She looked like she was going to be sick, and she went to the bathroom."

A few minutes later Amy reappeared. She was again sitting in the chair against the wall, but now she was holding a bucket up to her face just in case she got sick again. She later told me, "I booked it out of there I felt so sick." I giggled at how she told me she had gotten sick, but I knew how she felt. It was one of those times you just had to be there. We managed to find some humor in that situation. It wouldn't be the last time this happened to Amy, either.

It was nearly two weeks before I was discharged from the hospital. If it hadn't been for Amy meticulously documenting all the details along the way, I would not have remembered that by the time I was discharged I had had two heart biopsies, one vascath (of that one, I was well aware!) and four dialysis treatments. I only remember the very first dialysis treatment, and could not remember the rest.

The transplant was nearing. I was scheduled for two more weeks of dialysis, three times a week. I needed three plasmapharesis treatments and a Rituxan infusion. Rituxan attaches to the B cells, which make antibodies, and kills them. I needed to be suppressed as much as possible so my new kidney would not be rejected. It was a two-hour infusion that was given with anti-nausea medication and an antihistamine to prevent the most common side effects. Our plan to tackle this new treatment schedule started with us deciding to drive back and forth to the hospital for each of my treatments.

The vascath was an experience that came with several barriers to everyday life. It was very susceptible to infection, and the bandage needed to be changed immediately by a nurse if water penetrated through it. Showers were difficult. My arm was stiff and in pain. Trying to maneuver around the water spraying down was a challenge. It was a reminder of how much the little things in life can have such a profound effect. I couldn't move my arm higher than a couple of inches up from my side. That made it nearly impossible to wash my hair by myself. Embarrassingly, I had to ask my little sister to help me wash my hair even though I was twenty-five years old.

Before I left the hospital, we had both asked the nurse how we were supposed to cover up the vascath so it didn't get wet in the shower. She explained that there was nothing special to cover up the entire bandage. Other patients had used pieces of plastic zip-lock baggies taped together to prevent the water from getting in. Amy and I both looked at her and asked, "Does that work?" I couldn't help but think that cut pieces of plastic bags secured by adhesive tape would definitely not hold up in the shower.

The only way to find out was to try it. Amy and I cut and taped a lot of plastic bags to fit over my port only to have the bags slide off mid-shower. Each time we covered the vascath, the bathroom floor was littered with pieces of plastic baggies and paper tape. I now made record-breaking shower time. I was fast!

CHAPTER 27

One Headlight

"Hey, come on try a little.
Nothing is forever.
There's got to be something
better than in the middle"
—The Wallflowers

I had been home from the hospital only a couple of days. Things seemed to be back on track with the exception of finding a good way of showering with the port. March 26, 2009 was the new surgery date. Before that I needed to finish the final pre-op blood tests, consent signing and a meeting with the surgeon. We were heading down to the hospital to pick up my two-week calendar that detailed the tests and treatments during the final two weeks before the transplant. I had five dialysis treatments left and one, possibly two, plasmapharesis treatments, depending on my antibody levels. Amy and I also needed to have a few more blood tests each in order to finalize the cross-matching process. Before we left the hospital that morning, one of the transplant nurses told us that we needed to stop by Jane's office before we picked up our schedule.

We assumed that she was just going to go over what to expect from the meeting with the surgeon and the remainder of the time until the date of the kidney transplant. Jane walked Amy and I to a small room at the end of the hallway and sat us down at a round table. There were two other women sitting across from us in the cramped room. One was a patient representative and the other, a financial aid representative.

Jane sat down and, as she comfortably arranged herself in her chair, blurted out without even a moment's hesitation that the surgery was cancelled, again. It had now been cancelled for the second time. I looked at Amy with tears welling up in my eyes, as I had done so many times before. I was upset and angry. Amy looked Jane straight in the eye and asked, "Why?" Jane just sat back in her chair like what she was telling us it was not a big deal. She said that I was not guaranteed to receive Medicare. That information was contrary to what the person in the hospital's financial aid department had told Mom and Amy during my last ER visit, Jane had even called me to confirm it. It didn't make any sense that Jane was now saying that I wasn't guaranteed to receive the benefits to cover the transplant. I couldn't hold back my anger and was yelling at Jane as well as at the other two women who sat at the table. I must have repeated myself a dozen times yelling that I would be covered by Medicare and that my mom was working closely with Mark Kirk's office to get it approved as soon as possible.

The patient representative and the financial representative started talking but appeared to have no clue about the whole situation. They were ill-informed and came in with insufficient knowledge and a lot of misinformation. And on that basis, they were trying to stop the transplant once again. They tried to interject into the conversation a few different times, and Amy and I both told them they had no idea what they were talking about. The patient representative's office had already cleared this issue up the first time they talked to Jane. Amy and I were beyond upset.

Amy asked why they were stopping the surgery again. It couldn't have been just because I was possibly not going to be approved for Medicare. None of it made sense. Jane paused and then said that they had heard we were fundraising.

What I was thinking was, "You are going to stop the transplant because we are fundraising?" Jane continued to point out that we were not guaranteed approval for Medicare and that, if I did get it, they would take it away from me because we had been fundraising. They were attributing whatever money we raised as my personal asset. She also stated that we never told her that we were fundraising, and that was the reason for stopping. I didn't know we needed her approval to raise money to help with the cost of the transplant.

Not only had Amy's fundraiser been in the newspapers and online, she had told the patient representative about her fundraising efforts to try and cover the expenses. First, the hospital knew we were fundraising from the beginning because Ethan and Amy had talked to a hospital representative about it and how our story was going to the news outlets. And, second, how could the act of our fundraising be a valid excuse to stop a life-saving surgery?

I was so upset that I demanded that my transplant nephrologist who would be seeing me on a regular basis after transplant be paged to sit in on this little impromptu discussion we were all having. Amy interjected and explained for the hundredth time that the funds that were being raised were not personal assets of mine. They would go into my medical trust fund set up for me ten years earlier by COTA during the heart transplant (COTA was the Children's Organ Transplant Association that accepted funds for families and then pays transplant expenses by reimbursements through the individual's medical fund). The funds in my account were not my financial or other personal assets; technically, it wasn't my money, and neither I, nor any of my family, had direct access to it. It was strictly for medical expenses related to the transplants. It would help pay for medication and other expenses we couldn't pay for out of pocket.

Maybe if Jane and the other hospital representatives had asked about these things before we were invited to a meeting to be told that the transplant was cancelled again, we could have been spared this shocking and upsetting news.

My soon-to-be transplant nephrologist had made his way to the tiny room where he sat cramped in the corner. I told him he needed to listen to what was going on and that the way this was being done was not right. Too often the doctors don't really know what goes on with the patients aside from their check-ups in clinic. I was determined that he see what was going on. He sat in what looked like a state of minor shock. When I pressed him to say something all he could come up with is, "I don't know what to say, and it is what it is."

To this day, I can't understand how people who are supposed to be helping you can tell you that you will not get a life-saving transplant because you are fundraising to pay for the surgery. To top it off, Jane told us in her condescending tone that, "The kidney transplant is an elective surgery. You can live a long time on dialysis and insurance will pay for that." At that point I wanted to fly across the table and show her what it was like to "live with dialysis for an extended time." Amy had to calm me down and get me to stay in my chair. And yes, I just elected to have a kidney transplant and my sister donate her kidney. What was wrong with her? She was supposed to be helping, and clearly Jane was not helping. How do you have the nerve to tell a dying patient that the life-saving surgery is elective?

Amy asked Jane what we needed to do to prove that the money raised from our GiveForward fundraiser was not my personal asset in any way. She explained that Ethan would need to call or send a letter affirming that the money raised was not going directly to me. Someone from COTA would need to do the same. Jane didn't have a chance to finish her sentence before Amy got on the phone to call Ethan. I quickly called my mom, briefly told her what had just happened and asked if she could call COTA immediately.

This was the last time I was going to let Jane have anything to do with my care. I made it clear to my mom and Amy that I wanted a different social worker for the remainder of my care as well as for my future care with the transplant nephrology team. I guess it wasn't enough that we needed to go through another transplant, much less deal with another person who didn't know what the hell she was doing but was, in fact, quite adept at upsetting the patient.

The following article is evidence that the hospital knew that we had been fundraising. I understand that there might have been questions about personal assets when it came to the money raised. Yet, this last upsetting meeting could have been completely avoided by a simple phone call.

Article in the Chicago Sun-Times
Posted on 03/18/2009 by Ethan
Original article can be found at the Chicago Sun-Times website on March
18, 2009 by Maudlyne Ihejirika, Sun-Times Staff Reporter.

She makes sure sister has a chance to live

Jessica Cowin, 25, of Northbrook, needs a kidney transplant. Not extraordinary, except that she got a new heart 10 years ago. Jessica's sister, Amy, has managed her medical care for years. Also, not extraordinary, except the tenacious mother hen is only 22.

"Under hospital privacy policies, you can only have one other contact. For Jessica, it's me," Amy said.

Managing her only sibling's care includes serving as kidney donor and raising $24,000 in just over a week — through an Internet plea — after being told Jessica had to qualify for Medicaid before Northwestern Memorial Hospital would do the procedure.

Qualification can take months. Amy applied for Medicaid, but worried about waiting, she found GiveForward.org, a start-up Website providing an online fund-raising venue for any legitimate cause.

Her Help Jess page, at www.giveforward.org/helpjess, immediately set a record, and got publicity.

"Most of the donations came in small increments of $10 to $25 from young people around the country on Twitter and Facebook," GiveForward co-founder Ethan Austin noted. "It's pretty amazing."

Northwestern has now lifted the Medicaid stipulation and scheduled the transplant for April 2nd.

That's because Jessica's condition worsened, spokeswoman Kris Lathan said. Amy thinks it has more to do with media attention.

The transplant runs upward of $100,000. Jessica's current insurance pays a maximum of $30,000.

"We learned in November she was at end stage renal failure," Amy said, "In January, I tested to make sure I was a match."

Jessica first has to undergo a process to remove extra antibodies due to myriad blood transfusions, to lower her body's risk of rejection.

Boasting the nation's largest living donor kidney transplant program, Northwestern is one of two area hospitals offering the cutting-edge desensitization procedure.

But after the sisters completed prep procedures, the hospital said they'd have to wait on Medicaid.

"It is our policy to not proceed with transplant when patients have inadequate insurance coverage or have no avenue to cover the cost of the immunosuppressive medications," a March 2 letter explained.

"Suddenly, everything comes to a complete stop," said Jessica. "I was in shock. But Amy got working."

Amy directed donations to the Children's Organ Transplant Association (COTA). It accepts funds for families, who then pay transplant expenses and seek reimbursement. Funds unused go to other families.

When Jessica ended up in Northwestern's emergency room on March 3, Amy shared her story with the hospital's patient rep. Within hours, she was informed the transplant was to proceed.

"I want to make it perfectly clear money was never a deciding factor," Lathan said, "At the time she was referred to our transplant center, she had stable kidney functions. She was told to wait, get into the system. But as her health became of great concern, her physicians decided not to wait. It was Monday when the team met and the decision was made to transplant her with financial assistance pending. It was Tuesday she came into the E.R."

Jessica is currently on dialysis.

"I'm so happy we're finally going to get it over with," she said. "I don't know what I'd do without Amy."

Said Amy: "I love her more than anybody in the world. I just want her to be o.k."

CHAPTER 28

The Luckiest

"I don't get many things right the first time
In fact, I am told that a lot
Now I know all the wrong turns the stumbles,
and falls brought me here"
—Ben Folds

A classmate and good friend of mine, Alla, had talked to the mentor we had had as members of the Collegiate Entrepreneurship Club, DePaul Chapter. The year before I graduated, in 2007, I had been elected club president and Raman was our faculty advisor. Amy and I were regulars at the entrepreneurship center where Raman had an office. We spent many hours talking about our plans for our baking company and gathering advice from him and April who worked closely with him. I had not shared any of my medical history with him. Raman didn't know anything about it until Alla went to his office and politely demanded his advice. She spoke to him about how Amy was trying to raise money to pay for the remainder of expenses that would be incurred for the transplant. In typical Raman fashion, he jumped right in to help with this article he wrote in support of Amy, fundraising, entrepreneurship and social media.

> *How Twitter and Facebook Are Changing Fundraising*
> *Posted on 03/10/2009 by Ethan*
> *This story was originally posted on March 5th, 2009 in the CenterTalk Blog by Raman Chadha, the Executive Director of the Coleman Entrepreneurship Center at DePaul University.*
> *"1 Week. $21,000*. That's how long it has taken to raise that much money. In one week, a fundraising effort catalyzed, mobilized, and evangelized by social media has already generated over $21,000 in cash donations. All with no cost.*
> *If you have doubted the power of social media and social networking, I humbly ask you to stop doubting. If you have wondered, "What good does it do?" stop wondering. If you've asserted that, "It's just a fad," stop asserting. This story will hopefully change your entire perspective.*
> *Last Wednesday, one of my students approached me before class with the story that a recent DePaul University alumnus, Jessica Cowin, needed a kidney transplant. Jessica's sister, Amy, had volunteered to donate one of her own kidneys but the surgery bill would amount to $100,000. Of that amount, Jessica's insurance would only cover $30,000, leaving an incredible sum of money to be paid by a young woman and her family.*
> *So Amy did what any loving family member would do and should do—she reached out to her network and asked for help. She sent a Facebook message to fellow DePaul students and alumni sharing Jessica's story. She appealed to them to help out in any way they could. My student was one of those who received that message.*
> *Later in the day, Amy set up a donation page to, "Help Jess" at www.giveforward.org/helpjess (BTW, GiveForward.org is a Chicago-based social venture).*

She then created a Facebook page and invited, I imagine, all her friends to visit that page, learn more about Jessica's situation, and make a donation. Within a few hours, I had already received a couple more messages from DePaul students pleading for people to Help Jess.

So on Thursday, I visited the Help Jess page and made a donation. I was surprised to see that over $8,000 in donations were already made…in less than 24 hours. The amounts ranged from $10 to $5,000. It was amazing.

Then I started seeing messages on Twitter. Then I got more emails, Facebook messages, and Twitter replies and direct messages. I was watching the power of social media in real time and for a real benefit.

———

I made a donation because I know Jessica fairly well.

She was president of our Collegiate Entrepreneurs Organization chapter for which I am the faculty advisor. She launched a business with her sister, Amy, and worked with the Coleman Center to get it off the ground. (To this day, I'm proud that we were also their first customer.) She convinced her parents that their business could use some help, and so they, too, became a client of the Coleman Center.

Jessica would regularly stop into our office, with a smile on her face, chatting and networking with our staff, clients, and fellow students. You could find her studying in the lounge area outside our office on a daily basis. We all got to know her very well.

Yet, never once did Jessica mention her health issues, which included a heart transplant (yes, you read that right) at the age of 16.

In the middle of all that interaction, consulting help, conversation, and mere physical presence, Jessica never took it upon herself to draw that kind of attention. Her humility and modesty is an example for all of us, young and old.

———

But today, she needs the attention, and the power of social media has given it to her. Family, friends, and complete strangers have come together to save a life. But we haven't come together in a physical way. We didn't attend a fundraiser or have someone approach us at our homes or offices. These, "fads" called social networking and social media brought us all together.

They brought us together to make a difference in a span of time that is mind-boggling. And I'm asking you to continue this amazing effort, and to Help Jess.

Please visit www.giveforward.org/helpjess and help in any way you possibly can. Almost $50,000 is still needed to Help Jess.

A donation of any size will help us move towards the certainty that a young person's life can be saved. And after making that donation, tell your friends, family, and complete strangers to do the same. Use your voice, use your email, use your iPhone, use your Facebook, and use your Twitter.

Together, we can not only Help Jess, but we can Save Jess.

www.giveforward.org/helpjess

* Editor's note. Since this article was originally published Amy and Jessica's fundraising total has reached $25,626."

After this article was written, DePaul University donated one thousand dollars to my fundraiser and offered to publish our story in DePaul's quarterly newsletter, the *DePaulia*. This article was written just before we found out that the transplant was cancelled for the second time.

Everything was so up and down, stop and go that we couldn't keep up. At least I couldn't. I couldn't understand that money came before a life. After all, I did go to business school and knew full well that the hospital is a business and, understandably, needed to get paid for their services. But they are also in the business of saving lives. When it comes down to putting a price on a patient's life and well-being, something is wrong. Unfortunately, this is nothing new. Patients every day struggle to get the medical attention they need and is just out of reach due to a lack of financial stability and adequate insurance coverage.

Tuesday, March 17, 2009, had been probably the second longest day of this whole process. I have said before: shock doesn't begin to cover it. Instead, it was more like sheer panic. We were just about pushed off the edge of a cliff. It felt like we were free falling without a parachute. What do you do?

Amy and I tried to figure out how Jane, the lady from patient services, and the lady from financial aid could approach us. You are supposed to feel like you have a team behind you, supporting you and keeping you on track. We did not feel like we had any support from the team, much less from Jane. Once again, we took to our phones and computers, contacting everyone we could possibly think of. At the top of that list were the people in the media who were following our story. Amy and Ethan were great at updating everyone with every detail and this second cancellation of the transplant was big news.

 Less than twenty-four hours later, we received yet another phone call from the hospital, not Jane this time, telling us the surgery was back ON! I had no patience left for jokes and with an attitude I sarcastically asked if they were sure that this time the surgery was for real and how could I trust that they were not going to change their minds again.

It was real, and I finally had my last—and very official—transplant calendar in my hand. Only six dialysis treatments were left, three the first week and three the next week. I counted down at each session: "Five more to go. I can do this." There was finally an end in sight, and I was very grateful that I could now see it.

A few treatments in a row, I was seated one chair away from an older gentleman I had noticed there shortly after I started my treatments. He had noticed Amy and me, too, and struck up a conversation with us. Amy was finally able to sit in the dialysis lab without getting sick, as long as she didn't stay too long. The older gentleman asked why I needed dialysis. I briefly explained that I had had a heart transplant almost ten years earlier and the medication had become too toxic for my kidneys. I returned the question by asking if he had yet been listed for a kidney transplant. He sadly smiled and replied, "No." He went on to explain that his renal failure was due to years of living with diabetes and not taking good care of himself when he was younger. Amy and I smiled and sympathized with him, and I told him that I hoped his transplant would be soon. He asked when I was to have my transplant. I was confident to say that it was in two weeks. No more cancelled surgeries.

I smiled back at the older gentleman and turned back to watch the mini television that hung in front of me, conveniently attached to the back of the chair in front of me for optimal hours of viewing. I counted my hours in Dialysis by TV shows. Every hour-long program was another hour closer to the end of treatment. All I could think about was I just needed to get through six more treatments and twenty-four more hours of dialysis lab television, then I would never have to be there again.

CHAPTER 29

Counting Stars

"I feel the love and I feel it burn,
Down this river, every turn
Hope is a four-letter word,
Make that money,
Watch it burn"
—One Republic

M ark Kirk's office called my mom to tell her I had officially been approved to receive Medicare. It was cutting it close to the date of transplant, but it was done. I was headed down to the hospital for my first plasmapharesis treatment, and I was down to the last three dialysis treatments. My mom suggested that we stay downtown until after the transplant. Since I wasn't comfortable going to a dialysis lab closer to home, we had been driving back and forth to downtown for the last few weeks. It was more convenient to have all the treatments close to the hospital since we were at the hospital for weekly appointments, anyway. We figured that it was a good idea to stay in a hotel right by the hospital. I could walk to the remainder dialysis treatments and wouldn't have to get up super early to make it to my plasma treatments. It was nice because I was exhausted and didn't have the extra energy it took to get up, get ready, drive downtown, wait for treatment, get a four-hour treatment, get in the car and drive home. Just before one of my dialysis treatments, Amy and I ran around to at least four hotels within two blocks of the hospital trying to find last minute a place to stay for the next week.

Our final hotel stop was the Affinia Chicago. The staff seemed so attentive and accommodating of everything we needed. We had come in the front doors out of breath and quite upset with our previous attempts to find a hotel room. We explained that I was going to be on my way to dialysis treatments and, in just days, Amy and I were going to be having surgery to donate her kidney to me. The manager came out to personally show us to our room and to let us know that if there was anything at all we needed, just ask. We had a little time to relax; at least I did before I left for dialysis. The hospital dialysis lab was across the street and around the corner from the hotel. The walk there and back wasn't too terrible. Almost immediately word spread to the employees of the hotel that we were the two sisters getting and donating a kidney. Everyone asked us how we were doing the whole time we were there.

I had begun my plasmapharesis treatments that ran in length close to the time it took for dialysis. The plasma treatments were a little more tolerable. I tended to fall asleep for the majority of the time it took to run the machine. I had a really awesome nurse that always made sure I had everything I needed and that I was comfortable. I got distracted watching how she arranged the bottles she was going to use. She would pull out the plastic stopper that was in the top of all seven Albumin bottles the fluid that is replaced when the plasma is removed from the body, and line them up. Then she would arrange the tubes that were attached to the machine that connected to me and would lay them flat, untangling them when necessary. She gathered saline, and other bottles of fluids that, when each was empty, would be replaced until all seven were empty at the end of the treatment. She always asked me if I was hungry. I had free range on food and could eat during the treatments if I wanted to. Usually, I was so nauseated before, during and after that I didn't care to eat. The only thing that was consistent before every treatment was the chocolate milk from the cafeteria. That was the only thing that I seemed to tolerate. I figured at least I was getting some nutrition into my system, even if it was in the form of chocolate.

I was still very limited on fluid intake, which wasn't going to change until after the transplant. I could drink very little water, iced tea, pop, or anything. The more I drank, the longer the dialysis treatments would be because the more fluid they would have to remove from my body. I had gotten down to about 115 pounds and was all skin and bones. You definitely could see a difference from when I was at a healthy weight. If I noticed it, I know my mom, Amy and everyone else noticed it, too. I did my best to eat when and what I could although there was no promise it would stay down. Case in point, at my second plasma treatment I tried to eat a sandwich or mashed potatoes and corn (the only thing I craved other than the chocolate milk). This treatment was mid-afternoon and would take me well into late afternoon by the time it finished. So I tried to eat something. The nurse wanted to try and speed up the rate at which the plasma was removed and replaced. It was great for about a half hour. Then, I started getting light headed, felt tremendously sick and completely lost my sandwich.

I relate these situations not to scare anyone but to show that it wasn't a piece of cake and it's not just going in to see the doctor, sitting in the waiting room, waiting in the clinic room, checking out and leaving. And as insignificant as it sounds the impact was far greater. It wasn't the treatments that I remembered but everything else that contributed to it. I never really knew how to explain that until now. Sure, everyone's experiences are so vastly different.

CHAPTER 30

Tonight and the Rest of My Life

"Everything is waves and stars.
The universe is resting in my arms
I feel so light this is all I want to feel tonight"
—Nina Gordon

Alla was hosting an event at Enclave, a nightclub and bar, two days before Amy and I were going to have our surgeries. It was called the Blank Canvas Event, and green businesses set up tables to showcase their organizations. GiveForward was hosting a table there, and it would be the first time I would meet Ethan and Desiree. Our fundraiser page was going to be featured, as we were the first medical fundraiser they had on the site.

From the second we all met, we instantly connected with each other. I knew they were going to be in our lives for a long time. They are awesome, great, genuine people. The Blank Canvas Event turned out to include a lot of our friends from school. It was so nice to see and be with everyone. Even though

I didn't have much energy, it was important to me that I was there. The event was only a couple of hours before Enclave had to get ready for the nightlife of the city. Most of the group I had been so close with in college had come out to support Amy and me and to meet the team at GiveForward.

It was one of the last meals I would eat before the surgery, so we all went out to Gino's East for some of the best deep-dish pizza around the city. We were the most indecisive group, so it took us a while to decide what we wanted to eat. We pretty much ended up ordering nearly everything on the menu. I was happy being with friends. It took my mind off of the dialysis and all the drama that we had been dealing with at the hospital. It was nice to sit, eat pizza, catch up and act as silly as we did in college.

I briefed everyone on what the next few days were going to look like, right up to the time of transplant. It was going to be a busy weekend. We had the Shamrock Shuffle fundraisers, one more dialysis and a plasmapharesis treatment, then transplant. The Shamrock Shuffle was one of the most popular marathons in Chicago. It was held every St. Patrick's Day weekend and was a good opportunity to have another fundraiser. Ethan and a few of his interns set up a fundraiser the day after the Shamrock Shuffle at McFadden's bar to help us raise more money. They sold t-shirts and wristbands as part of a food and drink special. That fundraiser raised three hundred dollars more. From the beginning, this was more than just a fundraiser for Amy, me, Ethan and Desiree. We became friends. Ethan told Amy, me and everyone else that our fundraiser saved GiveForward from having to close their doors and give up on their dream of having this fundraising business, and in turn they saved us, as well.

We finally had everything in place. Medicare was approved and my last dialysis treatment was in a few hours. I felt like I could breathe, for once, without threat of the surgery being cancelled for a third time. My mom came down to the hospital so she could go with me to the final meeting with the surgeon, final paper signings and preparation information for the night before surgery.

Amy and I had been at the hotel for the last week. That morning, before I met Mom at the hospital, Amy and I enjoyed breakfast in the hotel restaurant. We both had coffee, I had granola, yogurt and berry parfait and Amy had almond French toast. We both had gone to our pre-op appointments a few days earlier.

We were told how to prepare for the surgery and what we were to do the night before. I will spare you most of the details, but one I remember was the day before we could not eat solid foods or anything that was red. I liked my cherry Jell-O, but that was out. We figured we would indulge while we could because the next day wasn't going to serve us up anything other than clear liquids or green Jell-O. No thank you!

Other instructions for the night before surgery were showering with antibacterial soap to make sure that we had as few germs on us as possible before going into the operating room. The night before Amy and I were to start our pre-op preparation, a friend of ours, Brandon, came by to see how we were doing. Amy and I were supposed to go to dinner with him, but it ended up being just me. That was great just to spend some time talking. Times like these make you realize how lucky you are and how lucky I was to have so many people around us and supporting us with everything that had gotten us to this point. That dinner took me away for a while and I was able to relax. Even though we ate right in the hotel restaurant, it felt like I was a million miles away.

I had had my last dialysis treatment earlier that day. I was so excited to get it over with and walk through the door to the elevator and never look back. I was told that because it was my last treatment, it could run about five hours in order to remove a little extra fluid before going into surgery. I did everything I could to talk my nurse out of letting it run that long. During treatments every week the doctors come by to check on all their patients getting treatment that day.

My doctor had been there for my last treatment, making his rounds. He came around and I made sure that my treatment was not going to last five hours. My time was just about over, and I had wanted to sit upright in the chair. All the chairs were oversized recliners, and usually I would lie back a little during treatment because sitting upright for over four hours was tough. Amy had come back in for the last few minutes of the treatment; friends and family were not allowed to stay with the patient except at the beginning and end of the treatments.

Amy had just walked back to where I was sitting and I explained, with a lot of excitement, that I was waiting for the nurse to come back and finish up with the heparin and to unhook me from the machine. I told Amy that I wanted to sit up, and before she could tell me, "No, wait until the nurse comes back over," I had already pulled the lever to move the chair into the upright position. I felt good, for about five seconds. Then I was overcome with a feeling of having the wind knocked out of me, and I couldn't breathe deep enough to catch a good breath.

Before I had time to think and before I had a chance to ask Amy to get the nurse, my eyes apparently rolled back into my head as I fell into the chair and passed out. When I came to, I had two nurses standing over me. One nurse had a wet paper towel and insisted that I put it on my forehead to keep me cool. The other asked me what happened. I unintentionally disregarded their questions and instead asked them where my sister was. She had been there a second ago. One of the nurses said that she had gone to the bathroom because she wasn't feeling good. The nurse asked me again what had happened. I told her that I wanted to sit up straight in the chair, so I did. I could tell just by the expression on her face she knew exactly what had happened and explained that was why patients were not supposed to move or change positions without someone there to help them. Sitting up too fast during or after treatment could make you lightheaded enough to pass out.

Oops, I guess that's what happened. I quietly sat there trying to recover from this little episode. I knew it was the last time I was going to be there and I was only minutes away from the final steps it took to release my vascath lines from the machine and walk out the door.

I finally found out that my sister was in the waiting room. I told the nurse that if she wanted to come back again, she could. Amy slowly made her way around the corner again to where I was sitting and pulled a little rolling stool over and took a seat. I couldn't figure out why she looked so pale. I asked, "Are you ok?" She replied, "When I saw your eyes roll back in your head and you passed out, I got sick to my stomach and had to rush out." I couldn't help but giggle about it a little. I felt bad that she had just witnessed that and it made her sick. We both laughed about it as we were reminded about the first time it had happened to her during my very first dialysis treatment. I guess we needed things to end like they started—with Amy getting sick! She had during that first traumatic dialysis treatment and then here at the last one I would need.

CHAPTER 31

As I Lay Me Down

"Though it's not clear to me every season has its change
and I will see you when the sun comes out again"
—Sophie B. Hawkins

I t was April 1, 2009 and I was officially done with dialysis. It had been nearly a month of tiresome treks back and forth to the dialysis lab, but I wouldn't have to think about it ever again. A week or so before the transplant, I had to be admitted to the hospital so I could receive the Rituxan infusion. Rituxan is used in the treatment of certain cancers, autoimmune disorders and transplant rejection. It aids in helping the B-cells prepare for, in my case, a new organ to be introduced into the body without immediately fighting against it and ultimately rejecting it.

It was a drawn-out infusion of two or three hours. The nurse couldn't use my port for this infusion. I told her she had one chance of getting the IV in and that was it. She used her one chance, and then she had to get another nurse to put the IV in the second time around. Standard procedures required I be admitted to the hospital for the duration of the two- or three-hour infusion so I could be closely monitored. This was because of the several life threatening side effects. These included, but were not limited to, serious liver, heart, and kidney problems and even death. Other less severe side effects were chills, itchiness, chest pain, shortness of breath, sleepiness and body aches or weakness.

Everything had, thankfully, gone smoothly. The Rituxan had no lasting side effects, I did not need a last minute dialysis treatment and my plasmapharesis treatments were over until after the transplant. Now, Amy and I were just hours away from surgery. We stuck to our clear liquid diet and all the preparations for surgery that night. Mom and Mike had come to the hotel to stay that night so we were able to all walk over to the hospital together. My father was going to meet us at the hospital at our call time, six o'clock in the morning.

Amy was the first to check in and would be the first to go into the operating room. All of us walked with Amy to the surgery check-in desk. I gave her a hug and told her I would see her later. I tried not to cry, I didn't want her to get upset or worry that I wasn't all right. Everyone gave her a hug and told her that they would be in her room as soon as they were allowed back to be with her.

I needed to check in on the transplant floor. We walked up there, and there was a room all ready for me. Amy was a couple of rooms down, and my mom, Mike and my father were going from room to room checking in on us and relaying messages back and forth between us. The nurse came in to tell me that Amy was heading to the operating holding room, and she would be heading to the OR shortly.

It seemed so surreal. We had fought so hard for this moment. I tried to take it in and relax. I was actually more relaxed than I thought I would be. The same calm that I had felt walking into the operating room for the heart transplant was here again as I waited for the phone in my room to ring telling me that it was my turn to head down to the OR holding room. I didn't talk to Amy before I heard that she had gone to the OR. I had only talked to her before, and we said our "I love yous" and "See you later" much like we had done nearly ten years ago when I walked in to my heart transplant. There was always that chance one or both of us wouldn't make it out of the OR. However, if we had been able to keep talking to each other, we never would have gotten to the OR that day.

About an hour or so later the phone rang in my room and I knew that was it. It was sitting right next to my bed on the adjustable tray table. My father was sitting with me, and my mom and Mike had come up to tell me that Amy was nearly done and she was doing really well. Even so, I asked the nurse while I had her on the phone how Amy was, and she reassured me she was fine.

My nurse that day and one of the people from the hospital transport team came into my room to wheel me down to the OR waiting room. I asked my mom again how Amy was doing and said that she had done great and everything went well and she would be heading to recovery in the next few minutes. As she was coming out of the OR I was heading in. The surgeon drew back the curtain and explained what he would be doing and how and where the incision would be made. Next, the anesthesiologist came in and told me that she had some good stuff for me before we went in to the operating room. My anesthesiologist was Dr. Childers, the sister of local Chicago news anchor Mary Ann Childers, and the attending doctor who would be in the OR with me. I thought that was pretty cool and then she asked if I was ready for some medicine and I said, "Yes."

My last memory was being told that Amy was in recovery and that she was the donor of a small kidney, laughing because I knew I could use that on her later. Then I gave my mom and everyone hugs and said that I loved them and that I'd see them later and to tell Amy the same for me. I was sitting up in the bed as the doctors wheeled me around the corner towards the two large stainless steel doors. I don't remember going through the doors or being in the OR, so I gathered that the medication had worked very well and quickly.

I woke up quite groggy back in the entrance of my hospital room. I managed to again ask where Amy was and if she was ok. My mom said she was doing really well. However, she was still in a lot of pain in the recovery area until they could get her a room. It took nearly ten hours to get a room for Amy so she could come back up to the transplant floor.

The nurses were talking to me now, explaining that they needed to transfer me from the gurney I came up on, back to my bed. There were a couple of nurses, I think, telling me step-by-step what they were going to be doing to get me into bed as fast as possible. The slightest touch or shift sent pain rushing everywhere. My back was killing me, and moving seemed to be impossible. It doesn't help when you have been lying on a metal table for hours with no pain control. That pain catches up to you quickly and never really can be relieved at that point.

They took hold of the sheet I was lying on, lifted it and put me in bed. It was the most painful thing I had felt in a long time. Surgery pain is very different from the chronic pain you eventually learn to deal with on a daily basis as I had done with my kidney back pain. Surgery pain is muscle pain and incision pain and it hurts a lot! I just yelled for the nurse to ask the doctor for some pain medications. She told me that she would go ask the doctor as soon as they got me back in bed and hooked up to all the monitors again.

My mom came in my room and told me that Amy was finally settled in a room a few doors down from me. She was in some pain, but the doctors already had her sitting up. It was amazing how fast they kick you out of the hospital after a transplant or surgery. The faster you are able to move around, the easier and better you will be able to heal from surgery.

The surgery was Thursday, April 2 and by early Friday evening, Amy was being discharged. Before her discharge papers were ready she had walked, slowly, over to my room and sat down in the chair that was just across the room. We just smiled and made sure each other was doing okay. We never really had to say very much because we always just knew by looking at each other how we felt. We joked about how Amy had a small kidney and how she was being kicked out later that day. I was being sent home the next day, but I needed to get the last two plasmapharesis treatments out of the way before leaving the hospital. One they did a little while after I had gotten back to my hospital room and the last was done Friday.

I saw my cardiologist, the surgeon, the transplant nephrologist, the social worker (that was the last visit I allowed her), the Walgreen's pharmacist that was in the hospital and another patient representative from whom I was able to get my discharge papers. There was a lot of finalizing all the details of my new medication schedule and instructions on what to do and not do after surgery. My antibody levels were low and stable and I was lucky to not need any further plasma treatments.

Saturday evening I came home to a houseful of friends and family who welcomed Amy and me home. I was tired and in pain, but grateful to be sitting at home. I had to sit with a pillow against my stomach to help with the pressure and pain. Moving bothered the staples that had been used to close my newest scar, but I managed. Many of my mom's friends from work brought meals over to the house so we didn't have to worry about dinners for a while. It was so very thoughtful and generous of everyone who did that for us.

CHAPTER 32

Follow Your Arrow

"When the straight and narrow gets a little too straight,
Just follow your arrow wherever it points
Say what you think, Love who you love,
'cause you just get so many trips 'round the sun.
Yeah, you only live once"
—Kacey Musgraves

My new kidney now sat in the front in my lower abdomen. The surgeon decided not to take out my diseased kidneys and there was no harm in that. The only medical reason for taking them out would be if they caused more problems, circulation or a blockage, than if they were left in. Eventually, what would happen is they would shrivel up and just be there "like two little prunes" because the surgeon had cut off the blood supply to them during surgery.

A week after the transplant I had my first kidney biopsy. It wasn't nearly as bad as I expected it to be, especially in comparison to the extravagant heart biopsies I had had. It still required a very large and long needle, but it was nothing compared to when I went in for a heart biopsy. It was performed as an outpatient test right in the office. I managed to get some medicine to relax before I saw the large, long, needle drawn from the plastic shell and inserted through my skin into my kidney. After two clicks of the needle, the biopsy was over. No lying flat on my back for six hours in a recovery room. I was able to move around freely after about an hour, as long as the bleeding was under control and my post-biopsy urine sample came back clear of blood.

I was hoping the doctors would remove my vascath the same day as my kidney biopsy, but they were unusually backed up with appointments and didn't get a chance to even look at it. I was more scared about the vascath being taken out than about having the biopsy. I was tired of trying to keep it dry in the shower and keeping the two lines from pulling when they got caught on my clothes. I was especially tired of the pain in my chest and arm.

I had three blood tests scheduled in the next few weeks and, for the first time, I had a home care nurse that came to the house weekly to check my blood pressure, listen to my heart, check the incision site for any abnormal spots, or discharge and to make sure my pain was under control. My recovery was progressing very well and the healing was faster than I ever remembered it being after the heart transplant. Even my home care nurse commented on the progress I was making in just my first week at home. Amy's recovery was quick and relatively painless, too. She had only a couple small incisions where the laparoscope and camera went in and sucked her kidney out for me to inherit.

A while back, I had talked with a friend about the possibility of playing on a softball team that summer. He was excited to get a co-ed softball team together and asked if I wanted to be on the team. Practice would begin in May, and the season would officially start in June and I was already planning on playing on the team. It sounded crazy, especially after having major surgery; I of course, made sure it was fine with my transplant nephrologist Dr. Friedewald before I officially became part of the team. His only request was that I make sure that nothing hit my abdomen where the kidney lay. I must admit that softball was a bit of a challenge. My body wasn't exactly at the point of being in softball shape. I couldn't run fast, couldn't dive for ground balls and had to avoid certain plays that would potentially hit me in the abdomen. The last thing I was going to do was go through another transplant because of softball! Granted, that was a bit farfetched, yet it was a possibility. The impact of a force like that could potentially damage my kidney, especially since it was just below the surface. Suffice it to say, I was careful during the two months I played softball.

As slow as everything seemed up until the point of surgery, it was lightning speed afterwards. A couple of weeks into my recovery I was desperate to get out of the house but couldn't drive. Brandon was the manager of a new, up-and-coming Chicago band that was playing at a new venue in the city. Going to see the band was a good reason to get out of the house. Amy and I invited Ethan out with us. It was the first time we had seen him since we had our surgeries. Even though the fundraiser was ending during the following month, our friendships with Ethan, Desiree and the GiveForward team were just beginning.

As my 26th birthday approached, I sat at home thankful for my life, my family, my friends and my future. I was back in the home that I had lived in for over 23 years—the home where Amy was born, and where there were memories of birthday parties, family barbeques, cooking experiments, marathon movie nights, the phone call for the heart transplant, and countless recoveries after tiring hospital stays.

It had been ten years since my heart transplant and a few months after I received my kidney, my second lifesaving transplant. Such life altering events put things into perspective for me. I realized that I could not have been luckier. I had a wonderfully loving and supportive mother, (step) dad and grandparents. I had a sister who constantly amazed me with her brilliant insights, intuitions and gut feelings. I was constantly asking her to tell me what she thought. Then there were all the wonderful, loving, and compassionate friends Amy and I share.

Everything was better than I had ever expected. I was feeling more and more like my old self, only a healthier version. I finally was able to fit back into my jeans. That was a big deal! I had only been able to wear comfortable yoga style pants that were flexible and cushioning to the scar more than jeans would have been right after the surgery. Plus, I couldn't button my jeans anyway because I was swollen, and the prednisone didn't help. It was an exciting moment when the time finally came that I could button and actually wear a pair of jeans out.

As much as things had changed, the more they had stayed the same. I had come off a lot of the medication in the first few months. I went from nearly sixteen pills to about eight every day. I had been put on Prednisone just as I had been after the heart transplant, but thankfully it was a far lower dose that would be tapered off within the first year after transplant. It took six months for me to completely eliminate it.

About four months after the kidney, I finally was given the "okay" to have the vascath removed. I was so excited and couldn't wait to make that appointment. It was one of the last things I needed to check off my list of things to get rid of. My blood count and antibody level was good and there was officially no need for further plasmapharesis treatments and, of course, no more dialysis treatments because my kidney was working perfectly. I had no idea what to expect when the vascath would be taken out. It was done in the office as a simple outpatient procedure, just like my appointments for biopsy had been.

There were a couple of nurses who started to prep me for the removal. A resident was going to be doing the majority of the work. I had had no idea it would be so detailed and so painful. I thought after they cut the two little stitches holding the vascath in place, they would just pull the rest out of my chest and I would be out of there. The nurse told me, "You will feel some pressure and a little pinching when they take out the two stitches." It felt like they were cutting my skin when they began to snip the stitches. It was not a feeling of pressure or pinching at all. It really hurt and felt like they had cut little pieces of my skin that, at any time, would start to bleed when they pulled and tugged on the tube and the two lines outside that were once used for treatment. I don't think my chest healed properly after they put that stupid thing in the first place. It was just as painful as the day I got it. The doctor did have problems removing the whole thing, and that didn't help at all. He and the nurse had to stop and let me have a break from the pain every few minutes. There was no way I was leaving that office with this thing still in me so I told them they needed to just finish as fast as possible. They continued to pull and cut and clean the area as they slowly and delicately went on. I was about to pass out because of the pain. Tears had been rolling down the sides of my cheeks, wetting the pillow beneath my head. The next thing I saw was the doctor pulling a long, thin, flat, white, and worm-like, flexible-material thing out of my chest. It was almost like watching a bad magic trick, where the magician pulls the handkerchiefs out of his hat or sleeve and keeps going on and on, with the audience wondering when it will ever end. I lifted my head to watch again and, finally, it was all over. The end of the flat tubing was completely removed.

The vascath was the final procedure and the last step I needed to get through to have the feeling of closure on the last seven months. It is natural to go through the emotional and physical ups and downs of any medical issue. It is part of the process, and is similar to the five stages of grief: denial and isolation, anger, bargaining, depression, and acceptance. Those five stages of grief are used in the context of losing a loved one but can also be felt and experienced during medical trauma.

First was denial and isolation. I was blindsided both times, first by my need for a heart transplant and then for a kidney transplant. Overwhelming emotions took over; there was disbelief in the news I was getting and in the realization of how this happened. My gut reaction was to say, "No. I am not going to do this."

Next was anger. It took me a very long to stop being as angry as I had been about my circumstances. I was mad at everything and everyone. I was mad at the IV pole and the sounds the machine made every time it beeped. I was angry at having to face another unknown and my family having to deal with it. That is possibly what made me the angriest—having to see them go through the pain of me being in pain.

Bargaining, number three, was interesting. I was always in this stage. I bargained with the doctors to wait on the vascath and dialysis. I needed to feel some sort of control and the only way I knew how to do that was to put in my two cents everywhere I could. I didn't have time to get a second opinion because time was short in both cases. I didn't have much time to spare when being listed for the heart transplant and was cutting it close for the kidney.

Depression was, is, perhaps the hardest stage to get through and it takes the longest to work through. I would often cry at night. When everyone was sleeping, I would pull the covers over my head and cry. It didn't matter what it was about.

The smallest thing would upset me, even if it was completely unrelated to my medical condition. Doctors who weren't listening, more tests to be done, getting sick no matter what I ate, it all added to the depression. I think in medical crises the depression lingers for a long time after everything is over with. I suppose that it is post-traumatic stress syndrome. It takes a long time for the emotional wounds to heal, not just the physical ones.

Last is acceptance, whether it's accepting the things you can't change or accepting that things are going to be okay. I remember when Great Grandma Annie died. She was one of the people with whom I spent many of my sick days. She would take care of Amy and me when Grandma and Papa were out. She was everything to me. I was nineteen when she passed away. I accepted that she had had a long, wonderful life and Amy and I had gotten to spend many years with her. Now, she was in a better place, without pain and suffering. Never again would she have to try and ask for a whole bottle of Aspirin, visit the emergency room or wake up in a place she didn't call home.

Sometimes acceptance is immediate and sometimes it takes a while. During the heart transplant, I was able to accept the process a little faster than I did with needing the kidney transplant. With the kidney transplant, I didn't I want to accept it when it was going on. There were so many roadblocks, and I was depressed and angry for the majority of it. I didn't accept it fully until the night before the transplant. There was no going back, no stopping the surgery at that point. It wasn't until then that I was finally calm and ready.

CHAPTER 33

Wonderwall

"Back beat, the word is on the street
that the fire in your heart is out
I'm sure you've heard it all before,
but you never really had a doubt
And all the roads we have to walk are winding
and all the lights that lead us there are blinding"
—Oasis

I don't think I would be doing justice if I didn't include the topic of insurance. Everyone needs it, but not everyone has it. It was something we constantly had to fight for and I probably will have to fight for the rest of my life. I guess I don't understand how lawmakers, politicians, and insurance companies can play with peoples' lives, controlling who is covered and who is denied. The insurance companies' bottom line means more than a life or, for that matter, more than millions of lives.

I still have panic attacks at the thought of insurance. There is no guarantee of being covered—especially when a person like me is considered "high risk," which equates to high cost payouts that the insurance companies just don't want to do. Granted, there is very little in life that is guaranteed, but I believe insurance should be one of those things. Everyone should be equally covered.

My sister was told she had a pre-existing condition because she saw a dermatologist. Something as simple as that could quite possibly affect her getting coverage in the future. Include cancer, heart disease, organ transplants and a multitude of other life-threatening conditions that will require medical attention and medication for a lifetime, you are surely going to have a hard time getting covered. As time goes on, this will be ever-changing.

Generally, people remove themselves from issues that do not directly affect them. It's true, at some point that we all do. We can't possibly deal with every little thing. Insurance is not a little thing. I recently found out that lawmakers in Illinois signed into law $1.6 billion in cuts in Medicaid coverage. Some people will be dropped completely from the coverage and the ones who are not will have significant benefit reductions. The prescription plans have been cut, as well.

Illinois is by far one of the worst states to get help with insurance coverage. The state and federal programs have all been significantly cut. Prescription drug plans are no longer sufficient (as of 2013) to help with the medication needed to survive, though the state funded insurance plans do allow up to four prescriptions a month to be covered. The only possible way to have insurance in 2012 was to have a job. Finding a job, at least in the economic state of 2012, was nearly impossible.

There is no guarantee that a person with a pre-existing condition will be covered, anyway, with some of the insurance assistance programs that the state offers because they have major requirements for being approved. Many say that you cannot be covered unless you have exhausted the Consolidated Omnibus Budget Reconciliation Act of 1985 (COBRA, a law that was passed by the U.S. Congress, signed by President Reagan, that mandates an insurance program that employees can opt into and use after leaving a job that provided health insurance) or have been denied with proof from a private insurance company. Another stipulation is the denial letter must state that you did not have any insurance coverage for nine months prior to being approved by the federal or state programs like the Children's Health Insurance Program and Student Health Insurance Plan (CHIP and SHIP).

I was able to receive Medicare during the kidney transplant because Medicare covers end-stage renal failure and the transplant for 36 months if you are an adult. After that, coverage ended. The anti-rejection medications alone cost over three thousand dollars a month and they are not optional. I know other patients have the same problems especially when they have pre-existing conditions. I suppose the only time, possibly, that you can get medical coverage is when you are very sick—or dying, as in my case—hence the Medicare program, but after you are healthy again you no longer need insurance? That is the time you need it the most. Yes, it is expensive for everyone. Most people cannot afford health insurance the way it is heading. Insurance companies are increasing the costs and cutting back coverage. It is a vicious cycle and it is exhausting, frustrating and upsetting. All the work you do to survive, go through life-saving transplants and treatments, seems to be worthless when you continue to have to fight for medical insurance. It is no wonder that people have to start fundraisers to help pay for the excess medical expenses, some that insurance don't even cover.

I found myself looking at some of the current medical fundraisers on GiveForward and almost started crying. Not only can I relate to the pain of how such medical issues affect the family, I also read that the fundraisers were due to extensive medical bills and lack of coverage. One was for a baby girl who had not been born yet, was diagnosed with a serious medical condition and couldn't get insurance to cover the surgery that was going to be needed after she was born. The medical coverage the family managed to get would only be temporary for a condition that is with the baby for a lifetime. Insurance has significant limitations, sometimes even when you have good coverage.

The Affordable Care Act that President Obama put forward and Congress passed still doesn't make coverage available to everyone. The eligibility guidelines still make it possible to NOT qualify; even when you have exhausted all other options and have done the best you can to follow all the requirements.

No one can afford not to be covered, even for one day. If something happens in that day of no coverage, you could be facing a significant amount of money

202 | the Hearts of a Girl

that would need to be paid to the hospital and doctors, or they could refuse service all together. What then? Are you left to die? And now, you have a pre-existing condition to add to that. Politicians on the other hand would say they are doing it to improve the future of healthcare and to save vital programs. In the short-term, it is a devastating move that feels like it goes unnoticed. People with the same circumstances that I have had to deal with will tell you the same thing. It is not enough we all have to fight to live, especially during serious illnesses. We have to fight for the very things that let us live. The saying, "If you don't have your health, you don't have anything," should be changed to, "If you don't have insurance, you don't have your health."

Finally, I am back to, "normal." I have had my fair share of typical relationships that didn't work out. I have cried over break-ups and have done online dating, and cried over that, too. I am just like any other girl who has cried over a guy more than once in their life. Of course, I dream about the man I will marry, what he might look like and how great and genuine he will be. My mom always tells me, "There is a reason why that relationship didn't work out. You have angels watching over you. When the right one comes along, it will be amazing!" I worry sometimes that, because of my medical history, the "right guy" won't come, but if they are the right one it won't matter to them.

In the end, I prefer not to be, "normal." It gets boring. I like excitement and adventure, and, in the last thirty years, I have had a good amount of it. I did have some relationships and many dates in college, both before and after my kidney issues. Just like in all my medical experiences I have also learned from my past relationships. It's part of life and growing, and it is important to be who you are and to do the things that make you the happiest.

CHAPTER 34

Bridge Over Troubled Water (Reprise)

"Sail on silvergirl, sail on by.
Your time has come to shine
All your dreams are on their way"
—Simon & Garfunkel

B ailey and I met on Facebook on a transplant page. Bailey was a heart transplant patient who was in need of another heart and a new kidney (it was her first kidney). She had made her hospital room her new home for several months while she was on the waiting list. I saw on Facebook that she got the call and was going to be heading to the OR for her heart first. Then next day they would do the kidney transplant. I texted her immediately as I had done so many times before saying, "OMG I am so happy for you! Stay strong! You got this." The transplants were a success, but her recovery was very slow. It was not how it should have been after receiving both organs. Her condition quickly declined. A few weeks later, she died in the hospital. When I saw the news about her, I ran upstairs and told my mom, barely able to get the words out about what had happened. I was in shock and crying probably harder than I have ever cried.

Before Bailey passed away in January 2012, she and I talked and texted each other regularly. She grew up very differently than I did. She was born and raised in a small town in New Mexico and then moved to another small town in Texas. She was always upbeat, even when she was having a bad day. We connected instantly. She told me that being from a small town, there was no one that she could relate to or talk to about her medical issues. Her friends knew, but they were now far away so she didn't get to see them regularly and she had a very limited support system. We had tentative plans to meet each other in person after her new transplants and once she was feeling better. She was going to teach me about ranch life and I, a city girl at heart, was going to show her around Chicago.

There were so many things she was enthusiastic about and that she wanted to do. She wanted to go back to school, write, have a boyfriend and get married—all things I could relate to. We talked about why guys were so confusing and if there would be that one out there for each of us. She talked about what it would be like to meet him and how she would finally be happy and in a good place as far as love was concerned. We laughed and joked and texted each other just to say hello or to talk about how she was feeling. I very much wish she was here to be able to experience it all. I know she would have given anything thing for that chance.

Everyone deals with significant disruptions in their own life very differently from the way I was raised to. I suppose it is a matter of how you deal and manage and push through it that makes life manageable. Can you really be normal and lead a happy life after such significant life-altering medical conditions? My definition of "normal" is one where my childhood was filled with doctors' visits and constant monitoring, tests, and checkups. My normal life will always be different from most other peoples', no matter who you ask. There are people who have grown up on a vineyard somewhere in California; there is another who grew up training for the rodeo. I guess my point is this: no one's life is normal compared to anyone else. They are all unique and should be embraced that way.

You can't compare. It took me a long time to realize that being unique is a gift. The only thing we can all relate to are those who have had similar experiences whether they are big or small, medical or non-medical.

On May 1, 2012 this realization hit me like a ton of bricks. Mom and I went to the premier party for a new documentary, entitled *The Heart of the Matter*. The Children's Heart Foundation founder and our friend Betsy Peterson had been instrumental in getting it made. As my mom and I walked up the curved driveway to the children's hospital, as we had done hundreds of times before, it seemed like it had all been a dream. And yet, the memories came flooding back. I hadn't been back to the hospital for nearly nine years and when I left, it was on a note that was less than pleasant. All the times we went to the hospital for my check-ups and tests and the heart transplant were back. It almost felt like I was doing it all over again. I had a rush of unexpected emotion that I thought had left me long ago. It was overwhelming, and just as we came up to the big automatic revolving doors, I felt like I was going to be sick. The comfort that I had once felt being there was now gone. So much had changed in the time since I was a patient there. From the outside it all looked the same, though the building was showing its age as I was showing my own.

The premier was across the driveway. I had never been on that side of the street before. Betsy and her husband Steve greeted us at the door. So many people from my childhood were going to be there. The doctors and surgeons who had taken care of me for so long and who had been a part of several of my surgeries were there. Dr. Weigel and Dr. Cole would be there, too, the two doctors who were like family to me. Being in that room with so many people who had gotten me to where I am now was unexplainable.

My mom pointed out Dr. Backer and a couple of the other doctors she remembered who were part of my team. She told me that Dr. Backer was the one who went to harvest the heart the night we got called to the hospital for the transplant. He had been there for my surgery, and he had done surgery on me previously. I had no idea he was the doctor who retrieved my heart. He looked familiar to me but he didn't really know me anymore, which brings me to this point. So many family members of the patient, as well as the patient, remember the people who were a part of saving their lives. The doctors are hard pressed to remember the patients, however. I am sure my one-time doctors knew me, but seeing me years later, in the present, must be weird for them to try and remember me from years ago. If I mentioned something about my heart, that would probably spark a memory for them more than my face.

In a weird way, I felt back at home. These were some of the people I grew up knowing. Dr. Cole and Dr. Weigel made it feel like I never left them, giving me hugs and catching up as we would do when my mom and I went to their office for appointments. This is where I fit in, where I had always fit in. I have a feeling these heart doctors do not see patients all grown up that often. In what I hope is the majority of cases, the patient grows up and moves on to see an adult cardiologist. In other cases, some patients do not make it into adulthood. And when they do, they do not often remember the doctors that helped them get there.

I was always very invested in the care I got and the doctors I saw, partly because that was how my mom had been. She had made sure to include me in all aspects of my care and explain to me the best she could what the plan was going to be. She always gave me a say in my care. After all, I was the one who knew my body the best and knew what I needed. In turn, I was able to form relationships with my doctors and remember them, the good ones and the not so good ones. It is just as important for us patients to see how it is for the doctors to see us all grown up and doing well. I hope that it makes them just as happy to see us as it does for us to see them. They had a hand in our survival and ultimately in our future.

What is happiness? I have always thought that I wanted to know what happiness is. I once believed that you could only be happy when you were doing something that kept you busy. The "something" that you needed to fill the time and help to do what you need to do to pass the time. But, then the feeling passes. One part of my happiness comes from being able to help others and by sharing my story. I hope that it touches one person, inspires one person, or helps one person get through all the unhappy parts that are the hospitalization, needles, tests, doctors, and the unknown. I only know that if it were not for my family and friends, I would never have truly been able to remember what it is like to be happy outside the dry, faded, white walls of the hospital. It is hard to go through a significant life-altering medical challenge such as a transplant, much less two, without your loved ones with you.

There was a patient I once shared a room with. It was only a brief period and I couldn't help but listen to him explain why he was in the office for his visit that day. I was getting my port bandages changed one afternoon to prevent infection before dialysis the next day. This other patient was there receiving treatment for a kidney virus (for which the treatment was another kidney transplant). He was on an IV when the nurse asked if he needed her to call any family members. He said that none of his family knew about him receiving treatments or that he had received a kidney transplant. He said, "It was better that way." Will he ever know what happiness is outside the hospital? I hope so. You are not ever happy in the hospital, you are happy when you get to leave.

Having left all that, I can focus on living my life, getting a good job, going back to school, one day getting married, and maybe having kids. It is not possible for me to carry my own children, but there are plenty of other options that I will discuss with my husband when the time comes. I had hoped to get back to thinking and dreaming about much of the future. You lose sight of those normal thoughts everyone has of what they want to do when they grow up. My thoughts were, "Just get through this and it will be okay." I never really had time to think about anything other than getting myself through these medical challenges the best way I could.

Now that I am in great health, it is harder for me to cope, at my very best, all the time with the normal things. I forget sometimes how much I have been through. Although it is not something I sit around thinking about. The ugly side to all this is that there is depression that comes along with it, whether it is during the diagnosis/treatment phase or years after. In my case, it has been after the fact that I find myself sometimes not knowing how to deal with normal life problems. I am so used to dealing with far worse and far more extreme situations that it is difficult for me to accept the normal parts of life.

This might sound crazy, but most if not all, patients go through some sort of post- traumatic stress. In my case I never had the time to stop and think about it until now. It was always there and I did have my moments where I was depressed about the need for a heart and then kidney. I guess I never really realized how hard the adjustment would be from being sick for such a majority of my life to having the time where I was healthy. The adjustment is rough and is going to take a long time. It is just another road that I have to figure out how to navigate. I guess that is what life is all about. I suppose it is better that I learn it now rather than later. It will not be easy; I just have faith that it will be worth the journey. I know it won't be a straight and narrow, easy, uncomplicated road ahead. For that matter, life for anyone isn't simple. You might have been blessed with the most luxurious life, but that doesn't make you immune to a life-altering medical crises. It is how you accept it and do what you need to do, make the strong choices that so many people don't.

I know some time, in the not so distant future, I will require another heart transplant. I do my best to try and live in the present and accept the things I can't change and try to embrace what I can change. I am doing my best to make a life for myself and I am very grateful that I have the chance to do it right now.

Life, to be continued…

Acknowledgments

"Life is too short to wake up with regrets. So love the people who treat you right. Forget about the ones who don't. Believe everything happens for a reason. If you get a second chance, grab it with both hands. If it changes your life, let it. Nobody said life would be easy, they just promised it would be worth it; value the people in your life who matter, have influenced, and made you. Not everyone is granted a second chance at something."

—Unknown

Amy. She has always had to deal with so much and has had to be strong for everyone else, leaving her emotions and needs on the sideline. It is hard for me, as her sister, to see her hurt, unhappy, sad or struggle with things. If anyone deserves everything, it is Amy. She has given up so many things so that she could help take care of me. The medical part never ended for her, either. She has saved my life countless times and has given me the greatest gift of all—her kidney. I sometimes wish the circumstances were different, that we had been able to know what it was like to have a normal childhood and not miss out on more normal times in our lives. Even so, I would not change any of my personal experiences or medical adversities. First of all, if I had had a more normal live, there would be no basis for this book. I wouldn't have the same passion and dedication that I have for organ donation, fundraising, and Congenital Heart Disease (CHD) awareness. I might not have the same closeness and love with friends and family.

Sometimes it is easy for people to forget what is really important. It is who you have not what you have in your life right now that is important. I struggle with this, as do Amy and my mom. I have seen the pain, upset, and grief in Amy as the years have gone by. Yet, she has never failed to be there right at my bedside in the hospital, at appointments or at home. I know she gets worried and scared at the slightest medical issue I might have, even if she doesn't show it, it is internalized. She is strong and unwavering and I would not have survived all this time without her. Both our futures are bright. She doesn't need to worry about living my medical life anymore. It is time for her to live her life and be happy. We will always be partners in crime and she is a huge part of the reason I am writing this book. She touches everyone she meets. We make a damned good team. I can only look forward to us pursuing our shared dream of opening a bakery and baking together, or going wherever life may take us. I look forward to seeing her fulfill her own personal goals and dreams because they will only be great. There will always be ups and downs in our lives. I will always be there for her no matter what. I can only leave my dear sister with these words by Henry David Thoreau, "Go confidently in the direction of your dreams. Live the life you have imagined." I love you.

Mom, you are my strength when I can't be strong for myself and even when I can, you still are. You taught me how to love unconditionally and to believe in my own convictions. Though you never planned on this type of medical life, a sick child and for a long time a single parent, you only inspire other parents going through the same medical issues with their children. You never missed a doctor's appointment, a single test or day that I was in the hospital. We argue when we agree and we laugh about it. Thank you for being my editor ten times over. I am proud that I am your daughter and that you are my mom. I love you so, so much.

There wouldn't be a story without the three organizations that saved my life; The Children's Heart Foundation, Children's Organ Transplant Association (COTA) and GiveForward.

The Children's Heart Foundation (CHF) gave us a loving support system and sense of community when we needed it the most. I was thirteen when we first sat down to speak with Betsy, the founder of the organization. It was from that point on, my mom, sister and I knew that they would be a part of our lives forever.

COTA came into our lives just as it was about to make a significant shift. I was on the transplant list and COTA was there to support us in the journey to getting transplanted as well as help us to fundraise to pay for the mounting medical bills. My medical trust fund is still in their wonderful hands and I know that when there is a transplant related expense I can breathe a little easier knowing that they are right there to help.

GiveForward is the third organization that literally saved me. From dedicated co-founders Ethan and Desiree, Amy and I were able to fundraise with them, raise awareness for medical expenses and ultimately get the kidney transplant I was in such desperate need for.

I cannot express how much love and gratitude I have for these amazing organizations. No words can ever express my deep feelings for The Children's Heart Foundation, COTA and GiveForward.

For more information on the organizations I am involved with please check out their website.

http://childrensheartfoundation.org
http://cota.org
http://www.giveforward.com

9 781630 477554